Reiki Healing for Beginners

Complete Guide to Heal Yourself and Others
With Reiki Including Energy Healing, Reiki
Meditation, Chakra Balancing, Aura Cleansing,
and Reiki Self Healing Techniques

Judith Yandell

TABLE OF CONTENTS

Introduction

Crystal healing is a practice that people have used for
I would like to thank you for choosing this book, and
I hope you find the information informative and
helpful, no matter what your goals may be. In this
book, we will be discussing Reiki and how to become
a Reiki practitioner. This book is not meant to be
used as a certification class, but it is a starting point
where you can begin learning about the practice and
working with energy.

Reiki has a very long history, and that is where our
first stop will be in this book. We will be going over
the history of Reiki and where it got its starts. This
will also go over how it works. That seems to be the
mysterious part of the whole process, which is
understandable given the fact that you can't see what
is happening.

Then we will move into looking at the connection
between your chakras and Reiki. Chakras play a big
part in Reiki healing as they are connected with your

internal organs. It's essential to understand what the chakras are and their meanings and connections to the body so that you can adequately work with Reiki energy.

After that, we will start to look at hand positions used in Reiki healing sessions. This will not go over actual healing sessions, only different hand positions you will want to become familiar with. Then we will look at some standard tools that can be used during a healing session. These tools aren't necessarily required, but they are beneficial, and many practitioners swear by them.

Next, we will look at the different Reiki systems. Many energetic systems can be used when performing Reiki healing sessions. Not every practitioner will use all of them, but it is essential to know what they are.

After that, we will look at how to cleanse the aura using Reiki. With a cleansed aura, you can spread positive energy and simply feel like a better version of yourself.

Then, we will go over how to cleanse yourself. This will go over different sessions you can do to heal various ailments you may be struggling with. These are only supposed to be used on yourself and not others.

That brings us to the last chapter, which will go over different methods of cleansing other people. You will notice that the hand positions and movements are slightly different since you aren't restricted in where you can move your hands like you are when performing a session on yourself.

Reiki healing is a great tool to have. It will require plenty of practice to ensure you are using the energy correctly, but once you get the hang of it, you will find that it can help you in many different ways. Thanks once more for choosing this book. Let's begin.

Chapter 1:
The Basics of Reiki

Most people believe that Usui Sensei or Mikao Usui was the one who created Reiki. Some believe that Reiki just applies to the method of healing that he created and discovered. When it comes to tracking down the origins of Reiki, we found that before Usui Sensei created his Reiki, there were possibly four other types of Reiki healing being used in Japan. This information was discovered by Toshitaka Mochizuki Sensei and Hiroshi Doi Sensei, who are two Reiki researchers.

A Japanese therapist, Katiji Kawakami, came up with Reiki Ryoho, a healing style, in 1914. He also published the book *Reiki Healing and Its Effects* in 1919 that discussed his Reiki healing. During this time, other Reiki healing systems were being used. These included "Senshinryu Reiki Ryoho," which was thought up by Kogetsu Matsubara, "Reikan Tonetsu Ryoho" which was thought up by Reikaku Ishinuki, and "Seido Reishojutsu" that was started by Reisen

Oyama. In March of 1922, Usui Sensei received the Reikie energy and created his own Reiki healing practice known as "Usui Reiki Ryoho." An interesting fact about the name he picked is that it shows he knew the other forms of Reiki Ryoho that had previously been used, and he showed that this new style was his. Due to World War II and all of the work performed by Takata Sensei, the other types of Reiki weren't used as much or stayed unknown during the time that Usui Reiki was being practiced and gaining popularity.

When thinking about what should be called Reiki, we have to think about all the other Reiki healing systems that were original and don't have any lineage that goes back to Usui Sensei. Most people believe that Reiki energy has been around for more than a thousand years. Then others believe it has been around since the beginning of time. Anybody can use Reiki energy, and many people have. Because of this, any system that makes use of Reiki energy can also be referred to as Reiki, and not just the forms that have roots back to Usui Sensei.

Because of everything that WWII caused, and the fact that Hawaya Takata and given Reiki to the West, Usui Reiki became the most commonly used form of Reiki around the world. By learning about Usui Reiki, you can develop a healthy foundation that will help you to learn more about Reiki.

The Usui Memorial

The best place to start learning about Usui Reiki is to look over the inscription on the stone erected in Tokyo in honor of Mikao Usui Sensei in 1927.

The inscription on this memorial dates back to 1927. It was written by Juzaburo Ushida, who was a student of Usui Sensei and a Shihan teacher. Usui personally taught him how to teach Reiki. He would also end up becoming the president of the "Usui Reiki Ryoho Gakkai." Another member, Masayuki Okata, edited the inscription. The English translation was done by Tetsuyuki Ono.

The large characters used in their writing system located across the top read: "Memorial of Usui Sensei's Virtue."

Mikao Usui

He has been called Usui Sensei by his students. On August 15, 1865, in the village of Taniai. This was near what we know as Nagoya today.

He was very interested in learning and studied hard. As he got older, he would go to China and Europe for his education. He studied religion, psychology, medicine, and divination. He ended up joining Rei Jyutu Ka. This was a metaphysical group that helped people to develop their psychic abilities. He held several jobs, including rehabilitating prisoners, a journalist, company employee, and civil servant. He eventually became secretary to the head of health and welfare, and he would eventually become the mayor of Tokyo. The connections that he formed during this job ended up helping him to become a great businessman.

All his experiences in life inspired him to move his attention to find the true meaning of life. During his search, he found a description of a state of consciousness that could give one an understanding of their purpose in life. It could also help guide the person to reach it. This was known as An-shin Ritsu-mei. Once a person entered this unique state, you would always be at peace no matter what was happening around them. From this place, one could complete their life's purpose. One feature of this is that the state remains without any effort from the person. Peace will just build up inside you spontaneously and is one of the different types of enlightenment.

Usui Sensei understood this idea on a much deeper level, and as such, he had dedicated his life to reaching it. This is one of the most important steps a person should take along their spiritual path. He discovered that this could be achieved by practicing Zazen meditation. He then met a teacher who taught him how to meditate. After practicing this for three years, he still hadn't reached the state he wanted to be in, so he found other guidance. This new teacher suggested another practice that required you to be willing to die to reach "An-shin Ritsu-mei."

When he learned this, he got ready to die. He went to Kurama Yama in February 1922. This was considered a sacred mountain located North of Kyoto. While there, he planned on meditating and fasting until he passed to the next world. Please understand that he wasn't trying to find a way to heal but was looking for a unique spiritual state. Even today, there is a waterfall Kurama Yama where people will go to meditate. To perform this meditation, you stand under a waterfall as the water flows over your head. This helps to activate your crown chakra. Some masters believe that he likely took part in this form of meditation. As more and more time passed, he got weaker. On the 21st day of his fasting, in March of 1922, a light came into his mind, entering through his crown. He felt as if lightning had struck him. He fell into unconsciousness.

When the sun came up the next morning, he woke up and realized that he no longer felt weak, and was full of vitality that he had never felt before. His ordinary consciousness was replaced by high-frequency energy, and he had a new level of awareness. He was filled with joy to realize this.

Once this happened, he was excited and raced down the mountain to let his Zen master know what had happened. While he was running down the hill, he ended up hitting his toe and falling. Like any average person would do when this happened to them, he wrapped his hands over the hurt toe. As he did this, he could feel the energy flowing out of his hands and into his toe. It wasn't long before the toe stopped hurting and his toe was better. He was amazed. He realized that he hadn't just had an illuminating experience, but he had also received a gift of healing. He then and there that his purpose in life was to heal and teach other shows to do the same.

He moved to Tokyo in April 1922 and began a society he called Usui Reiki Ryoho Gakkai. He opened another clinic where he gave treatments and taught a class on Reiki healing.

It started as nothing more than healing energy, but he would soon create the Reiki healing system. This happened in 1923 after the Great Kanto tsunami and earthquake that damaged a large portion of Tokyo. This ended up injuring and killing thousands of people. Since many people needed healing, he decided to speed up training his new teachers.

He created many of his techniques like Seishin-to-itsu, Gyoshi ho, Reiji-ho, Byosen scanning, and Gassho. He also created an attunement method that made it easier for other people to learn Reiki. Before this, the methods he used to teach his students about Reiki was to hold their hands and give them the energy, but this took too long. The Reiju kai helped to make this process a lot faster, and there were several methods that he used. He also created Reiki symbols.

He gave many different attunements to his students. He didn't just give them one set. The reason behind this was so that his students could develop and refine their abilities so they could channel Reiki energy. This helped to make the energy used more versatile, and it allowed him to heal more conditions in less time. There isn't a limit to the effectiveness and quality of the energy that a person can channel.

The demand for this was so immense that Usui Sensei's work grew more prominent than his clinic. This led him to create his larger clinic in Nakano, Tokyo. Due to this, his reputation spread across Japan. This was when he began to travel to treat and teach others. During this time, he taught over 2000 students and appointed 20 teachers.

He received the Kun San To award for all of the work he did to help others. On March 9, 1926, as he was traveling to Fukuyama, he had a stroke and died. He has a grave a Saihoji Temple, but some people believe that his ashes were hidden somewhere.

Chujiro Hayashi

Before Usui Sensei died, he contacted Chujiro Hayashi to start his clinic to spread the power of Reiki. Usui Sensei liked that he had worked as a Naval doctor. Hayashi quickly started to create a school that became known as "Hayashi Reiki Kenkyukai." After the death of Usui, he left the Gakkai. The Hayashi clinic was in Tokyo. He started to keep in-depth records about the conditions and diseases that his patients came in with. He also noted which hand positions worked best when treating certain illnesses. He came up with *"Reiki Ryoho Shinshin"* based on all the records that he kept.

They only used the handbook if a practitioner couldn't use Byosen scanning to figure out which hand position they should use. Most of his students received their training through hands-on experience in the clinic.

Hayashi transformed the ways that Reiki was done. He moved away from the patient sitting in a chair to them laying on a table. Several practitioners would heal them at one time. He came up with a better system for Reiju. To help his students get more training while traveling, he created a new way to teach Reiki. He would teach both Okuden and Shoden in one seminar that lasted for five days. Every day would have two or three hours of teaching with one Reiju or attunement. He encouraged all of his students to regularly receive Reiju after their classes ended to refine their Reiki.

He took a trip to Hawaii and lived there from 1937 to 1938. This was before the Japanese attacked Pearl Harbor. When he returned to Japan, the military asked him to give them information about the locations of military targets and warehouses in Honolulu. He wouldn't do it, and they declared him as being a traitor. They made him "lose face," which caused him and his family to become disgraced, and society ostracized them. The only thing he could do to rectify this was to commit seppuku or ritual suicide. He honorably died on May 11, 1940.

After he died, his wife Chie Hayashi ran his clinic for several years, but she soon retired. Since he or his wife didn't appoint anyone to take over his clinic, it came to an end. Some of his students might have tried to teach, but nobody took over his clinic. Somebody found that Chiyoko Yamaguchi Sensei was a student of Hayashi and still practiced Reiki well into 1999. People encouraged her to start teaching what she learned, and she did. She died in 2003.

Hawayo Takata

Hawayo was born on Christmas Eve in 1900 in Kauai, Hawaii. Her parents had immigrated from Japan and worked in the sugar cane fields. She ended up getting married to a bookkeeper on the plantation where she worked. They had two daughters, and he died suddenly in 1930 and left her to raise their children alone.

She worked extremely hard to provide for her children and didn't rest much. She developed a lung problem and abdominal pain and soon had a nervous breakdown. It wasn't long before her sister died, and she had to travel to Japan with her body to be buried. She thought she might be able to get help for her health problems in Japan.

After going to the funeral and speaking with her parents, she checked into a hospital. She was soon diagnosed with asthma, appendicitis, gallstones, and a tumor. They told her she needed an operation, but she wanted to be seen at Hayashi's clinic first.

She was not familiar with Reiki, but she was impressed that their diagnosis was close to what the doctors had diagnosed her with. She started getting treatments. She would get treated by practitioners every day. The heat she experienced from their hands was so intense, and she thought they had been using some type of equipment on her. She noticed their large sleeves and grabbed one of them to see if she could find what they were using on her. She didn't find anything. After she said what she was trying to do, he laughed and started to explain about Reiki.

She started to improve, and after just four months, she was completely better. This made her want to learn more about Reiki and start healing other people. She moved back to Hawaii and began practicing Reiki. She created several clinics. One of these is located on the Big Island. She would initiate new students and provide them with treatments. She soon became well-known and took a trip to the mainland to teach people about Reiki and offer them treatments. She proved to be a mighty healer who said that she was successful because she did quite a bit of Reiki on her patients. She would often do multiple treatments, and these would sometimes last for hours so she could treat difficult cases. She would do these for months until her patient was better. She would sometimes teach her patient's family so they could work on the patient, too.

She changed up how she taught since the original Japanese teachings were too hard for the Western people to learn. She developed her hand positions that she called the foundation treatment. This had eight hand positions that were on the head, shoulders, and abdomen. She would also add in some places for the back if needed.

The most important thing you need to know about Takata Sensei is that Reiki would not be known today if it wasn't for her. At the end of WWII, Japan was, pretty much, at the mercy of the US. One of the conditions the US placed on Japan was all types of healing had to have a license to practice. Some obtained their license, but the "Usui Reiki Ryoho Gakkai" didn't want to be under the control of a licensing board and went underground with their practice. They made sure not to talk to anybody outside of their group, and they would only practice Reiki on one another. This made it more difficult for other people to learn about Reiki. Since they couldn't trust new members, their Reiki died when they died.

However, Takata Sensei lived in Hawaii. This meant that she could continue teaching Reiki, and kept it alive. She was a fantastic teacher and ended up teaching several classes all over the mainland and

Hawaii. Before she died, she appointed 22 Reiki that has helped to carry Reiki into the modern world.

Reiki Evolution

There aren't any limits to the possibilities that Reiki offers. Reiki is meant to be developed and changed with the times. This holds for the techniques that a person uses in Reiki, but the healing energy will always remain the same.

Reiki's energy comes from an infinite source. It does not matter how it has been developed, or how it evolves. The person using it will always channel a portion of the energy through the body that is still available. The effectiveness, quality, and benefits of a person's energy can improve over time.

This was explained by Usui Sensei when he told his followers that he would never reach the top of the Reiki healing system. He said he would always be one step under.

How Reiki Works

At its basic level, Reiki treatments can help to remove stress from the body. A person doesn't just move toward their balance in spirit, mind, and body. Depending on their level of physical health when they started Reiki, their body's healing mechanisms will start working better.

How does Reiki release tensions to help their body heal? This question still hasn't been answered. While there is documented evidence of the effectiveness of Reiki, like increased immune health, lower stress hormones, lower blood pressure, and lower heart rate, there are only a couple of theories as to why it works.

The body's quick response to Reiki suggests there is a complex process that engages various systems throughout the body at the same time that shifts the body from being dominated by the "fight or flight" response to a more relaxed response. This supports the body's healing mechanisms. Some scientists believe that Reiki's spiritual, emotional, mental, and physical healing gets triggered on a subconscious level that they call a biofield.

What is a Biofield

This is a medical term created for the intricately layered energy field that surrounds and penetrates our bodies. This is an extremely subtle field, and there hasn't been any scientific technology that can say it exists. For more than a thousand years, the prescientific, indigenous, traditional medical system has recognized a balanced, pulsing biofield as the foundation to our well being and health. They see a disturbance in this balance as the start of an illness.

The healing traditions of indigenous cultures from all over the world use vibrations to return balance by drumming. Instruments, like the tamboura and the didgeridoo, as well as humming and chanting, are used to bring balance into the body. All types of vibrations that come from music and sounds are supported by science. People believe the healing during a Reiki session happens through the kinds of vibrations.

One theory says that the Reiki healers carry an energetic vibration that the patient's body responds to. Reiki effects can be seen when the patient's attention shifts to the wellness they feel inside themselves. You can then be able to understand Reiki as training the patient to be conscious of their health. This works like how a grandfather clock will change to the rhythms of another clock in the room. This is the same way we can relax when we are with others who are in a state of deep peace. Reiki connects the practitioner to a feeling of inner peace, and it doesn't matter how we are feeling at that very moment.

Most therapies try to restore balance within this biofield. Yoga, shiatsu, qigong, and acupuncture are just a few. Reiki seems to be the most subtle of these that balances the patient by subtle vibrations instead of manipulating the body even in the gentlest way. Reiki may be closer to meditation than other therapies, but it doesn't come from within the biofield but comes from a subtler source that physicists have given the name of the unified field.

How Reiki Relates to Other Therapies

Reiki has been described as an alternative and complementary practice that uses energy fields to change a person's health. Reiki practitioners have found that Reiki is different from other therapies and is a lot closer to meditation. While most treatments use specific techniques to access a person's biofield to make specific corrections, Reiki practitioners don't diagnose, and they don't reorganize a person's biofield.

Reiki is a very passive practice. The practitioner's hands are very still for most of the treatment. They only move to change the placement of their hands. They will be neutral. They won't make any attempt to fix their patient or to change their biofield. They don't control Reiki energy. They only rest their hands just above the patient's body.

Reiki energy arises spontaneously to a person's need for balance at any particular time. By doing this, treatments are designed with the recipient in mind, although the practitioner might use the same sequence of hand placement for every treatment.

Reiki is usually given as a full body treatment but could be done in an abbreviated therapy for a specific area of the body. In emergencies, Reiki can be very soothing.

Chapter 2:
Chakras And Reiki

With a basic understanding of the history of Reiki, let's take a look at some of the more technical aspects. Reiki gives us the ability to transfer tranquility within us, helping to heal the mind and body. Chakras are the little spinning wheels of energy centers that live within us, which carry a considerable responsibility to emanate energy to keep our body and mind functioning the best that it can.

While it can be easy to lump the use of chakras into the "new age" world because of how popular they have become, it's important to remember that chakras have been a thing long before the New Age movement got a hold of them. Within the Yogic tradition, the body contains seven energy centers, known as chakras. When the centers are open and healthy, we are too. We find openness in our mental, physical, and emotional lives, as well as within our relationships with others and ourselves. When these centers become blocked due to illness, injury, or disconnection from others, we can feel that blockage within us. It can often leave us feeling frustrated, stuck, and as if we lack vitality.

During our childhood, we learn certain things that place constrictions in our chakras. For example, if we are repeatedly criticized for the way we sing, we may close the fifth chakra, limiting our ability to speak up for ourselves.

Negative experiences, fears, and trauma can cause imbalances within the energy system that will manifest into challenges like disease, stress, anger, or insecurity. We will often use psychology to better understand ourselves, which is a great thing to do, but we usually leave out an important thing, our energetic system. We not only should address our psychological issues, but we should also manage our underlying energy system, which can affect how we express ourselves, live, and breathe.

This is where energy healing helps. Energy healing supports our energy systems by removing constrictions that have been placed on them. How can we tell if our chakras are balanced?

The body is continuously in a state of flux between imbalance and balance. Balance isn't static and is always moving. Awareness is the best place to start that will help to bring attention to your mind and body. This enables you to learn your body's clues and signals. You will start listening to your body on several different levels, and it will serve as your guide.

When you start feeling happy, right, and relaxed in the world, then the energy is flowing correctly, and we feel as if we are inflow. However, when we start to feel stressed, anxious, or depressed, then it means our energy has become depleted, and our vitality levels could be affected as well. Over time, this will affect your wellbeing, and this where Shamanic or Reiki healing comes in.

It seems as if the pace that we are supposed to keep continues to get faster, to the point that we feel as though we have to be going 24/7. As we continue to push ourselves forward in life, many of us wind up losing harmony and balance.

We often don't choose to be grateful for the things we have and enjoy the day. We all end up worrying about the future or the past, and we allow the present to move right past us. All of this worry and stress affects our energy, and thus it blocks our chakras, preventing our energy from flowing freely.

A block within your chakras is an area in which your energy is constricted or trapped. When dealing with one of these blocks, you have to get your energy moving, which is what Reiki does. Once you get the energy moving again, your body will create harmony and release imbalance. Reiki can help to align your chakras.

Not a single chakra works independently of the others. They all work together as part of an energy system. Each chakra can only work to its full ability when all of the other chakras are engaged.

Each chakra has its role to play in balancing certain areas of our lives spiritually, mentally, physically, and emotionally. There are quite a few things that can affect the chakras. This can be anything from our emotions or mental conversations to our physical environment. It is imperative, if you want to remain in the good health, that you become and stay aware of how unbalanced or balanced those chakras are.

Energy

Our life force comes from our energy. We have to make sure we have that energy if we want to reach the things we desire. The more energy we have, the better off we end up feeling, and the greater chance we have of getting the things that we want. In Japan, this is known as Ki, which means universal life force. Energy is always flowing through our body, and in several healing aspects, it is viewed as moving through our chakras, even though we can't physically see them.

There is some of the energy that we can feel, but the majority of it is unconscious. I want you to take a moment and let your eyes close and think about the last time you felt joyful, such as watch the sunset. Notice how you feel when you bring this moment up in your mind. You might notice that you have started to smile, your heart feels warm, or you feel peace in your tummy. Now, take a moment and think about a time when you were facing a challenge or struggle. Notice how this feels within your body. You could notice that you feel tight in your chest, your palms start sweating, your heartbeat speeds up, and you feel anxious.

Did you notice the big difference between those moments? When you were thinking about that moment that you enjoyed, you felt relaxed and inflow. However, when thinking about the challenging situation, you felt upset, tense, and out of the flow. You react this way as your body responds to the energy and thoughts.

Simply put, if you only think about a challenging thing, you will find yourself tired from trying to figure it out. You could even start experiencing anger or a knot in the pit of your stomach. From here, you find it a lot harder to make choices that are going to help your greater good.

Energy wants to move, but it can get stuck. Healing will help the energy to continue moving so you don't wind up getting lost in your mental dialogue or emotions.

The Seven Chakras

Traditionally speaking, there are only seven chakras. However, some people believe that there are 12 chakras. These chakras are believed to be located above the crown chakra. The most important thing is to understand the seven main chakras. Once you have those figured out, and you feel moved to do so, you can start to work on the other five if you want.

1. Root Chakra

The first chakra is the root chakra, and it is located right at the base of your spine and creates your energetic foundation. It is depicted as the color red. This chakra represents earth and is connected to your survival, such as protection, food, and shelter. This chakra stimulates your need to remain healthy to stand up for yourself to ensure you survive. This is where our need to be connected and grounded comes in. Ideally, this chakra provides us with security in our life. It shows us what we need to survive. It grounds the spirit in the physical world.

On a physical level, it is connected to the bones, and the colon, anus, prostate, gonads, and adrenal glands. The adrenal glands are the primary organ that humans need for survival as it produces and releases cortisol, which controls our fight or flight response. The adrenal glands also have a connection with the third eye.

Fear is one of the primary energies that can significantly affect the root chakra. When out of balance, you start to experience anxiety. The anxiety is most commonly connected to the fear of change, fear of moving forward, and the fear of abandonment.

2. <u>Sacral Chakra</u>

The second chakra is the sacral chakra and is found in the lowest part of the abdomen around the sexual organs. Its color is orange. The chakra is closely connected to Water, as well as our sexuality and emotions. The function of this chakra is to ensure you have a sense of self and that you get to experience your inner child. This is where our inspiration and creativity resonate. It controls your need for sensation, whether that means sight, touch, taste, sound, or smell. Ideally, it should bring you the ability to accept change, feeling, and sexual fulfillment. It opens us up to the things that we desire and allows us to revel in the delight and beauty of life.

On a physical level, it is in control of the womb, ovaries, and menstrual cycle, as well as the male sexual organs. It is also connected to the moon, which helps regulate menstruation and fertility. This is why the sacral chakra is often seen as a feminine chakra. It's also related to the low back, so you may experience low back pain when this chakra is not balanced.

Guilt is one of the primary energies that can significantly affect the sacral chakra. When unbalanced, your guilt will become unmanageable. Intense guilt can wear a person down, making it difficult to express their emotions. This can cause you to avoid family and friends, give up hope, and feel miserable.

3. Solar Plexus Chakra

The third chakra is the solar plexus, and it is known as the power chakra. Found in the middle of the abdomen, near the bellybutton, the solar plexus chakra is yellow and provides you with the energy of enthusiasm, power, and heat. This is where you find your autonomy, personal power, will, creative expression, decision, and metabolism. When balanced, you experience self-worth, confidence, self-esteem, and can make decisions that bring you to align with yourself.

On a physical level, it is related to the digestive system, pancreas, gallbladder, spleen, and liver. When this chakra is balanced, it helps with the production of insulin.

Shame is one of the primary energies that can significantly affect the solar plexus. When unbalanced, a person starts to question their self-worth and drive. Shame can significantly affect the body by slowing down digestion. It can also bring about negative relations with food.

4. Heart Chakra

The fourth chakra is the heart chakra and is lies in the middle of your chest. It is the seat of your compassion and love and is the color green. The chakra helps connect the lower chakra, or physical self, to the upper chakras, or spiritual self. This helps to be our love and draws things into our lives that we love. When balanced, it allows us to feel centered, at peace, compassionate, and to love deeply. It will enable us to love ourselves unconditionally.

On a physical level, it relates to the blood and oxygen circulation, the function of the lungs, breast, upper back, sternum, and heart. These areas are significantly affected when there is an imbalance.

Grief is one of the primary energies that significantly affect the heart chakra. When left unbalanced, it can create more suffering than we can handle, leaving us with longstanding sadness. Love is vital to the health of this chakra.

5. Throat Chakra

The fifth chakra is the throat chakra and is centered in the throat and is the color blue. The throat chakra is what gives you your creativity, self-expression, and communication. As you begin to learn more about your authentic and individual self, the throat chakra allows you to express yourself, and share what you need. It frees up our communication so that we feel happy and centered. It also helps when we spend time meditating to connect to our high self to gain guidance. This is most closely related to your inner self and is closely connected with the soul, and gives you the chance to listen when the soul speaks.

On a physical level, it relates to the upper lungs, windpipe, ears, parathyroid gland, thyroid, and neck. When unbalanced, you can experience problems in these areas, like a sore throat.

Dishonesty is one of the primary energies that significantly affect the throat chakra. A lack of integrity and lies are also negative aspects of this chakra. When unbalanced, a person could either feel as though they can't speak up for themselves, or they could turn to be deceitful or lying.

6. <u>Third Eye Chakra</u>

The seventh chakra is the third eye and is located in the middle of the brow. Its color is the color indigo. The primary function of this chakra is inner vision. This is where your soul knowledge and intuition lives. This is where you can open up your spiritual and psychic awareness. When it is balanced, it gives you knowledge and insight. The third eye chakra shows you the power of your mind. You can use this to help you dream big and create the reality and life that you have always wanted.

On a physical level, it relates to the central nervous system, cerebellum, pituitary gland, brain, eyes, ears, sinuses, nose, and face. You could experience problems with any areas if the third eye is unbalanced.

An illusion is one of the primary energies that significantly affects the third eye. A lot in the world can dazzle us, but we have to see them for what they truly are. When the third eye functions correctly, we can distinguish between what is right and what is false. It allows us to perceive the world accurately.

7. <u>Crown Chakra</u>

The last chakra is the crown chakra, and it is located at the crown of your head. The crown chakra is purple and is the center of your consciousness. This is also what gives you access to the greater consciousness of the world, allowing you to connect to the world as a whole. This is where your soul comes into the body when you are born and where it exits when you die. Once you have developed and balanced this chakra, it can bring your harmony, spiritual connection, understanding, wisdom, and knowledge. It helps to awaken us to divine beings, connects with the divine, and helps us experience being one with everything.

On a physical level, it relates to the cerebrum and pituitary gland. It can cause headaches when not balanced.

Attachment is one of the primary energies that significantly affect the crown chakra. When a person creates a negative attachment to a person or object, it is often due to boredom, alienation, depression, an inability to concentrate or learn, and confusion.

Clearing Chakras

Yoga, Reiki, and acupuncture are some of the most common ways to clear out the chakras. When the chakras are blocked, the energy flow in a Reiki session won't be able to flow through the body as it should. That's why it's essential to work on unblocking the chakras before healing specific ailments. These practices can also help to uncover and release emotional issues.

Every stage of our development leaves behind mental conditioning that creates our views. Often, these learned patterns, perceptions, and behaviors don't serve us well. When this occurs, our programming connected with each chakra, with the root chakra connected to our childhoods, has to be consciously recalled and reprocessed to experience growth.

During energy healing, people will experience an emotional clearing after, which often results in a temporary intensification of the problem before a permanent relief from it.

Chapter 3:
Reiki Hand Positions

A Reiki session consists of a practitioner placing their hands on or over the client's body with the intent for energy to flow. There is no complicated ritual that takes place during a healing session. The only thing that happens is an exchange of energy between the client and practitioner with a shared intent of healing. According to Reiki teachings, Reiki energy is smart and knows exactly where it needs to go and what it needs to do. The practitioner allows the energy to flow without trying to direct the energy. A simple intent will cause the energy to flow, and that intent will produce the energy.

Treatment Protocol

There is a traditional protocol that is taught to practitioners that involves different hand positions. The positions are spaced along the client's body, and when used together, they provide coverage of the body. While the energy is placed where it is needed most, it is understood that the energy stays close to where the practitioner's hands are placed. By making sure you cover all of the body evenly, the treatment will be the most effective.

These positions work similarly to "training wheels." Once you have gotten used to using Reiki, you can feel free to experiment based on what you think you or your client needs. There are hand positions for both the front and the back of the body. Behind the neck, heart, kidneys, and sacrum are significant positions for Reiki.

While the hand positions are simply a guideline, some Reiki Masters will insist on just using only the hand positions. Most practitioners make a point of developing their intuitions that helps to guide their hands to where they need to be during each session. One of the most common ways is the sweep, where the practitioner sweeps their hands through the energy field, looking for any hot spots. These hot spots show areas that need extra healing energy.

There is one note I would like to add about body privacy. If you plan on performing Reiki on others, it will require you to place your hands very near or on body parts that many people view as private. Since the point of Reiki is to fully heal the body, it is best not to leave those areas out during a treatment session. Some people need their private body parts healed. At the same time, you also have to deal with privacy and the risk of abuse. Make sure that you professionally perform your work.

Every practitioner has come up with their way to deal with this. It is best to inform your client and get their verbal permission before your session so that there are no surprises. You have a couple of options that you can use when it comes to dealing with the private areas that won't involve touching them. First is to ask the client to put their hands on their body, then you can place your hands on top of theirs. You can then "beam" the energy through the client's hands. Another way to do this is to simply hold your hands over those areas, without touching them, and beam the energy from a distance. Lastly, you can also use distance healing techniques.

Another vital thing is practitioner comfort. A full treatment has been known to last upwards of an hour. Depending on how you position the client, it could put stress on your body. This is why you should not have them lying on the floor. It is best to have them in a chair or on a table, like a massage table. This is both comfortable for the client and the practitioner.

The Basics

The basic hand positions are the ones that can generally be expected to be used during a first treatment, as they are the most commonly used positions. Each position is meant to help balance the energy in an area and get rid of stuck energies in that space so that you can start to relax, lower stress, and create space for the body to heal and function better. Reiki is done with a very gentle, static pressure from the practitioner's hands on the traditional areas or with their hands hovering just a few inches over the body. Reiki works the same whichever way the practitioner chooses to do things. Once again, the practitioner will not touch private areas. With that in mind, here are the most commonly used hand positions.

Position A – The palms are lightly placed on the forehead, or their hands could gently cup the eyes.

Position B – The palms are soothingly placed around the sides of the face and temples.

Position C – The head is cradled in the hands of the practitioner.

Position D – The hands are placed around the throat or jawline.

Position E – The right or left hand may be placed close to the neck or right above the collarbones, while the other hand hovers over the heart chakra.

Position F – Hands are gently placed upon the upper abdomen.

Position G – The hands are placed near or on the solar plexus or mid-abdomen.

Position H – The hands are placed near, or on the mid-lower abdomen, just a few inched under the bellybutton.

Position I – The hands could be placed on the knees, ankles, or feet. These are optional positions and are only used if the practitioner feels that this could benefit the client. They could also choose to move onto hand positions on the back.

Position J – If the client is on a massage table, the practitioner may ask the client to turn over onto their stomach with their head in the face cradle or resting on one side. The hands are then placed on the area of the shoulder blades.

Position K – The hands are moved down to the area just below the shoulder blades or mid-back.

Position L – The hands are then moved to apply gentle pressure on the lower back.

Once all of the primary positions have been performed, and all stuck energies have been balanced or removed, the practitioner might move their hands over the body using a sweeping motion to cleanse out the energy field of leftover energy debris.

Self-Healing Positions

Learning how to heal with Reiki is a unique process. That's the way most Reiki masters will tell you to practice solely on yourself at first until you have learned the feel of how to heal and work with the energy.

I want to reiterate for a moment that intention is essential, so the first thing you need to do before you start a session, whether on yourself or another, is to declare your purpose of sending light through your hands. This is going to help activate your energy flow. Another way to do this is to rub your hands together to start the flow of energy. Better yet, do this while stating your intention.

Once you have reached a second or third degree of attunement, you can activate the energy through Reiki symbols. You will eventually start being about to feel when your palms can be moved, but having them over an area for around ten minutes or so is usually enough.

For the following positions, they will be broken down into leading positions and secondary. The leading difference is the parts of the body they are used for. For example, the main positions may be the head, heart, or kidneys, while the secondary are the knees, shoulders, or soles of the feet. Also, you can slightly adjust these positions to use them on another person, but the goal is to practice them on yourself first.

- Main Positions

First Position – The top of the head.

This is where energy enters your body. You start here to help develop a stronger consciousness and to help clear out the pathway to create a strong connection with the Divine and your true self.

For this position, place both of your hands on top of the head.

Second Position – Low head and between the eyebrows.

With these positions, you are cleaning out the energy to activate the memory, wisdom, intuition, and center of intelligence.

For this, you are going to be placing one hand on the lower back of the head and then placing the other hand across the forehead.

Third Position – Palms over the eyes.

Our eyes are polluted with images every single day. By sending energy to the eyes, it will help you to perceive things better.

For this position, hover both hands, one over each eye.

Fourth Position – On the ears.

Our eyes are also polluted with numerous sounds and information every single day. Cleaning out the energy centers of the ears helps to balance the brain hemispheres.

For these positions, rest either hand over your ears.

Fifth Position – The neck area.

Self-expression and communication are vital for a happy life. Therefore, sending energy to this space will help you in various ways, including communication rather than merely talking.

For this position, place one hand on the back of the neck and the other hand at the neck's front. You can also put both hands on the front of the neck.

Sixth Position – The middle of the chest.

We have all built up several emotions within us, some of which need to be removed. Using Reiki here can help to open up the heart in the right way.

For this position, carefully place one hand behind your back, resting it in the middle of the upper back. Place the other hand, over the heart. Alternatively, if you can't reach one hand behind your back, you can rest both hands over the front of your chest.

Seventh Position – The solar plexus.

This is considered the center of protection. Cleaning this area will help strengthen your inner security, and it helps to energize the organs in this space.

For this position, carefully place one hand behind your back, resting in the middle of the back. Place the other hand, over your stomach. Alternatively, you can place both hands over your stomach area.

Eight Position – The naval area.

About an inch below the belly button is the center of ambition, sexuality, and creativity. Healing this area will help you have healthy relationships, make you feel more comfortable with yourself, and socialize.

For this position, carefully place one hand behind your back, resting it along the low back. Place the other hand, over the lower abdomen.

Ninth Position – Kidneys

Healing this space will not only help the navel area, but it helps to increase vitality and energy. It can also help to heal and sustain the organs.

To perform this position, you will rest both of your hands on either side of the low back. They should be placed in the area where the kidneys are.

Tenth Position – The sacral area

This is located in the inguinal level. Healing this place will improve your grounding, strengthen your body, and vitality.

For this position, hover both of your hands over the private areas.

- Secondary Positions

The Shoulders – This is where the initiative and emotional centers of energy live. When we hold a lot of emotional "baggage," the shoulders will often become very stiff and tense. Cleanse this space will allow them to relax.

For this position, cross your arms over your chest and let your hands rest on your shoulders. You can also raise your hands and rest them on the back of your shoulders.

The Hips – We tend to have desires and emotions that are often left unexpressed. Cleansing this space gives you a feeling of peace.

To perform this position, you will place your hands on the front of the lower abdomen, one hand on either side. This is in the area of the hip bones.

The Knees – We tend to have physical tension in this area most of the time. We can all agree that we hold a lot of pressure in this area that needs to be cleaned out and relaxed.

For this position, work one knee at a time, place one hand behind the knee and the other on top of the knee.

Fee and Soles – We walk a lot every day, and we pick up the energies of those places. We then bring that energy home with us, and it starts to accumulate. Cleaning here helps to balance the inferior body segments and allows us to ground correctly.

To perform this position, work on one foot at a time, and place a hand over the top of the foot and the other underneath the foot.

Techniques To Enhance Treatment

Some techniques can be used during sessions that improve the process and enhance the hand positions. These techniques are beaming, scanning, cleaning, and tapping.

Beaming represents the idea of sending light to something or a person. All you have to do is hold your palms up to send Reiki healing energy to your desired situation or person. To help amplify this effect, it is best to visualize that you're sending out a beam of light from your hands.

Scanning can be used on yourself or another person. As you hold your palms one beside the other, slowly move them over the body, from head to toe, to search for different vibrations. The feelings you notice can differ from person to person. The sensations you may feel are stinging, pulsating, tingling, cold, or warmth.

Cleaning is a technique that is rarely written about but is very useful. Basically, after a treatment, you will use your hands or simply visualize brushing any negative or residual energy out of your energy fields, sending it out and into the ground. This should be done slowly, with no rush, for your entire body.

Tapping is a more pointed way to treat a person or yourself. It is a great way to unblock and purify different spaces in your body. All you have to do is use a rhythmic tap, using your fingertips on the affected area. You may not want to use this everywhere, but the thymus gland is an excellent example of where you can use tapping.

One last thing that is not exactly a technique is swiping. This follows treatment. All you have to do is use your right arm to swipe up the left arm and the left on the right. Do this three times for both arms. You can do this for the upper body as well. Take the right arm and swipe, starting at the left shoulder and finishing at the right hip. You will then take the left arm and swipe from the right shoulder to the left hip. This helps to get rid of any residual energy that may have been left behind during the session.

Chapter 4:
Common Tools

Learning about the tools you need to bring healing to others and yourself is required if you want to have a healthier and better life. These tools are a part of Reiki. This is a straightforward but powerful system that you can use.

Reiki healing used along with the tools listed below will help you bring vitality and health to all parts of your life, from your DNA cells to the broad reach of your spirit and consciousness.

You can use Reiki to help heal yourself on a karmic, quantum, mental, spiritual, and physical level. These tools you will read about are energetic "add ons," and will deepen and enhance the crystal's capabilities. They are straightforward and simple to implement.

You can start using these tools today to jumpstart your healing. Let's take a closer look at these tools you will be using and how you can use them to supercharge your healing.

People who practice Reiki healing will create a relaxing place for their sessions. They will set the mood by dimming the lights, playing some meditative music, or have a bubbling water fountain. Below you will find some tools, attire, room furnishing, and other tools that Reiki healers use.

Reiki Portal

In traditional Reiki, special symbols are used to send the energy out. While these aren't typically called a portal, in reality, that is what it is.

By using Reiki, you can use that portal to send Reiki through space and time, but you can use it to bring in healing energy from other places in reality and the universe.

When you have learned this technique, you could use Reiki to make a portal located about six inches above your head that will connect you to the realm of Angelic Healing. You could make a portal near your spine to get aligned to Diving Healing or whatever your needs might be.

You could have a certain kind of energy that allows you to connect to a specific spot on the planet. It might be a powerful spot such as the Vortexes in Arizona. You can connect with the energy of these places through your Reiki portal.

All of these portals could help you create a deeper level of healing. You can use them as a stand-alone technique or in combination with other self-healing.

Reiki Laser

This is a powerful, direct, and quick method. It is a concept that was referred to as the Reiki Cord. Reiki Laser is an extremely concentrated beam of light between any point in space and time.

You can use it on a karmic, emotional, or physical level. Since these sessions usually are very intense, you should only do them for a couple of minutes, so you don't overwhelm yourself or whomever you are healing.

This is the perfect tool to use when healing through time. You might have injured yourself ten years ago, a year ago, or last week. You can invite Reiki to make a laser that flows through you to that point in time.

Just remember to ask Reiki to get rid of any lasers that have been created after a couple of minutes.

Reiki Hologram

Making a Reiki Hologram is a great way to shift your energetic signature into an organ system or an organ itself.

To do this, you will need to ask Reiki while you are relaxed to create a hologram for one of your systems like your respiratory, skeletal, digestive, or muscular system or an organ to help it function at its highest level of healing and health. Then you will ask that hologram to merge with a place inside your body, a specific organ, where healing is needed.

This usually is used when deep healing is needed. This tool is useful when you can't sleep or are restless. You could create a hologram in your nervous system or brain as an alpha wave.

Reiki Meditation

Reiki meditation uses Reiki to change various meditative states within your healing. You need to use it to supplement your ordinary healing practice to take your healing to a deeper level.

The best thing about this tool is that it lets the crystal do all the work after you have invited it to bring you into a meditative state for inner peace and stillness.

You can do this right at the end of the beginning of a basic self-healing session. You can also feel free to use this at any point during the practice if it feels like you should.

You could use it to bring yourself into a state of self-love or meditation. It could be used to take you into meditation, where you will experience the deep love that the Divine has for you. You will be experiencing the exquisite fullness and beauty of the Divine Love.

Your Reiki could affect your meditations on a cellular level. Think about a part of your body that might need some healing. You could invite Reiki to bring some cellular consciousness into that specific area into a meditative state to express vitality and health.

This is very essential since diseases can come from various thoughts or emotions held in specific places within the body. You can use Reiki to change this consciousness.

All you have to do is visualize healing a specific disease possibly before it has had a chance to even manifest through a loving, gentle, and simple process. Reiki doesn't need you to revisit or find the root of the problem. It has its divine intelligence. It knows where it needs to go and what it needs to get rid of even if you don't.

Combining Reiki with Other Tools

Whether it is hypnotherapy, Shamanic Reiki, Crystal Reiki, Angel Reiki, meditation, color therapy, pendulum dowsing, or other things, Reiki practitioners might combine Reiki with different types of treatments to give their patients the best outcome.

To know which one to use and what to combine them with, keep reading.

Reiki Stones

These aren't your typical tools used by Reiki healers. Instead, they are a set of tools that have been engraved with symbols. Reiki symbols can help increase energy and can direct the flow of chi. The four main Reiki symbols are the symbol of connection, harmony, power, and master. They are great for absentia Reiki that can help seal your intent while helping you focus.

Shamanic Reiki

If you naturally connect to nature, the spirit world, the elements, you might want to try Shamanic Reiki. Meditative journeys are performed to visit your spirit animal, ancestors, or spirit guides to strengthen their sessions by bringing you messages or healing from them.

You will use a drum, rattles, chants, songs, whistling, and invoke the elements and directions to make a sacred place.

Reiki Cards

Every card has a specific purpose and a technique that you can use to achieve a particular goal. The "Listening Card" gives you strategies that help you talk to your higher self. The "Freshen Up Card" offers you a sound, breath, and exercise method that will revive your energy while purifying the body at the end of a long, hard day.

Divination Tools

Using pendulums are typically taught by most Reiki masters. By using pendulums, you can detect energy and find answers to any questions that you might have.

If you infuse the pendulum with your Reiki energy, it will balance your chakras and get rid of any blockages and pain. Making sure you have a crystal pendulum is better since the healing energy won't get blocked by metals.

If you want to get accurate answers to your questions using a pendulum, you have to ask your questions so that they have a "yes" or "no" answer. You could also use tarot cards, runes, or I Ching as your type of divination.

Reiki Pendant

This isn't a physical tool you use, but a talisman for you to wear to invoke the ki energy. The symbol of Cho Ku Rei can be used as a switch to turn on your Reiki energy.

Ho'oponopono

If you use this in your daily life, it could create miracles. This is a very ancient technique. It can free you from any sort of negative emotions or destructive patterns that you might have picked up.

It doesn't require any formal training or being initiated by a teacher. You can use it to heal yourself, and if it is recommended as homework from a therapist, you will see results immediately.

Massage Table

This is the best tool when you are doing Reiki treatments. You can special order a table that is a bit wider and more padding to keep your clients comfortable. But these modifications will make the table a lot heavier for you to carry. If you will be moving your table often, then a standard table would be best.

Candle Rituals

For this type of Reiki, you just need a sacred space, an intention, a candle, and a clear visualization about what you want. You can use different color candles for a specific task. Let's say you want to clear away negative energy and some protection. You should use a white candle. If you do Reiki regularly, candles can automatically tune into your intentions and won't require you to preprogram them.

Reiki Amethyst Pendulum

Pendulums can be used in energy medicine to measure a person's energy level and help find imbalances in the person's energy field or chakras. Pendulums can also be used as a divination tool. You can program the crystal to help heal. Pendulums with or without a crystal can be charged with Reiki energy.

Crystals

Crystals can be potent tools that you can use for manifestation and healing. To use a crystal, you just have to clear it of any programming and then give it a new intention. You can create a crystal grid that will amplify its energy to be directed toward a specific situation or goal.

Different crystals could be used for a particular type of task. Putting an amethyst crystal could help you sleep better.

Reiki CD

There is a vast variety of Reiki music out there for you to choose from. Play these during your Reiki sessions to help relax your clients. Music is an excellent complement to any healing treatment, and you will never go wrong with playing music in the background.

Essential Oils

Depending on which scent you decide to use, aromatherapy could treat depression, trigger healing, trigger a memory, act as an energy agent, brings pain relief, helps relieve stress, and it can relax you. It could be used as an antibiotic in some cases.

A couple of drops of orange essential oil can eliminate your daily stress to help relax you.

Reiki Poster

You may want to think about having a poster that features the basic Reiki symbols on the wall of your healing room.

Past Life Regression

If you want to access a past life experience or memory, get rid of a painful experience, confusion, or negative emotions, you need to try past life regression. When you can understand why your life had to be the way it was, all the negative karma associated with the experience and the pattern that kept repeating itself will be gone. Reiki can bring this experience to life and give you awareness and protection while accessing these uncomfortable situations.

Reiki Magazine

This is a news magazine that contains articles on all the aspects of Reiki. It is a quarterly publication and is 72 pages long.

Vision Board

Using a vision board, you can find your goals and focus on manifesting these things without getting distracted. Sending Reiki to your vision board and drawing Reiki symbols on the back of it will speed up the process.

Reiki Hand Poster

This poster shows the 12 basic hand positions for doing a Reiki treatment.

Intuitive Guidance

Some practitioners will offer intuitive guidance as a part of their session. This method will use intuition to bring messages to your patient. If you set an intention, a helpful message might happen when you send Reiki energy to your patient, which could help the healing process.

If you have psychic skills, like telepathy, clairsentience, clairaudience, or clairvoyance, they act as part of your intuitive guidance. The more you practice Reiki, the better your gift will get.

Pyramid Reiki Timer

This timer has eight settings that you can set it to so that it goes off at certain intervals. The intervals can be set up to 90 minutes. This can be a helpful tool to use as it can remind you to move your hand placements. The timer has a quiet signal and can be used by any kind of healer or therapist to help regulate sessions without watching the clock.

Color Therapy

Each color has its frequency and healing properties. Try this: visualize the color yellow during a Reiki cleansing or cover yourself with yellow Reiki chi balls to attract success in your career, increase personal power, and improve digestion.

Reiki Books

There are several books on the market about Reiki healing that you can use as a textbook. Most beginners can use these books to help start their learning process. It can help any Reiki practitioner to deepen their Reiki wisdom.

Violet Flame

If you have persistent blockages or patterns or need some deep healing, this powerful tool could be used. It can help turn blockages into a light, but it could act as a source of power, protection, and strength.

It doesn't matter if you decide to do a violet candle meditation, violet flame breath, or violet flame bath; you won't be able to ignore its healing abilities. Once you have been attuned to it, its effectiveness will be even better.

Water Fountain

Water fountains have a way to make the room calmer. They can be used in any room you want to bring a little more relaxation to, like the kitchen, home office, recreation room, or bedroom. There are many varieties for you to choose from.

Angel Reiki

Angels can add a Divine touch to your Reiki healings. Their help during a session or using an angel card reading can seal the whole process. Every archangel or angel will have its responsibilities and tasks.

If you need healing, you can call on Archangel Raphael. He is the supreme healer in the Angelic realm. They can't step in whenever they want, as this interferes with free will, so that means you have to ask them for their help, otherwise they can't step in.

Reiki T-shirt

Some T-shirts have the principles of Reiki printed on them to help remind you to follow the Reiki creed that all healers are taught. Clothing that has been adorned with Reiki symbols or words is a great "uniform" for you to wear when doing sessions. Wearing your Reiki shirt around is a great way to start a conversation with others who want to learn more about Reiki.

Synchronicity is communications that lovingly come from the universe, so if any of the tools or techniques speak to you, you should try them. Energy is always woven into synchronicity.

The longer you practice Reiki, you will become more aware and will be ready to try other tools that could add some extra zest to Reiki.

Chapter 5:
Reiki Systems

There are several different Reiki schools, and within each of them, they have their masters and teachers who like to explain things in their way. Some provide attunements to their students from their viewpoint, and then others stick with the old Japanese Reiki traditions. So which is right?

All of them are right, and we will look at why.

Reiki is split into different levels. Reiki started as one whole thing. Reiki didn't start out having a systemized way of being taught, and there were no levels or degrees. That's why we have to understand some important things before we go any further into this.

Reiki was given to us from a higher plane of existence through Mikao Usui, a Buddhist priest. This is why Reiki fits very well into our physical world because there is way more than we can see. The spiritual, physical, and energetic worlds fit together like a puzzle. We, humans, are the ones who chose to make the separations to have a clearer understanding of Reiki. In reality, these separations don't exist. This brings me to my next point.

Every Reiki level has its purpose. The separations don't make one level weaker than the next. It is a more straightforward path for us to understand things and learn Reiki. There are even Reiki Masters who have a lot to learn, and there are level one practitioners who have fully integrated with the philosophy of Reiki.

After Mikao Usui receives his calling, he turned to his fellow monks for advice. That's when he decided it was time to travel to Mount Kurama, where he started a ritual of meditation, prayer, and fasting. Once his 21-day fast came to an end, he experienced a vision that left him completely exhausted. It was this vision that told him about Reiki. After he returned home, Usui Sensei healed people. They were interested not in just receiving Reiki, but in learning how to do it as well.

Therefore, he ended up having many students. One of them was Chujiro Hayashi, who then trained Mrs. Hawayo Takata. These three people are the reason why we still have Reiki today.

During the Second World War, Reiki would have become extinct had it not been for Mrs. Takata. She managed to bring Reiki to the West, with some help from Hayashi Sensei. During this time, Reiki was split into different degrees. The main reason for this was to help students have a more linear and gradual evolution.

There should be no rush in Reiki. We all have to take the time to absorb new information. We need to study, understand, and then use the information. This is why everybody has to take the time to adapt to the new energy in their body. We all have an optimum rhythm that we operate on. Therefore, we have to make sure that we thoroughly learn information before we start using it.

If we rush things, we run the risk of overwhelming our minds with information, which will drain our bodies of energy. It can be a lot harder to repair this damage. That's why it's best to take some time to learn and move closer to your goals slowly. Every Reiki level represents an energetic and spiritual leap towards a new level of consciousness, awareness, and knowledge.

Back in the day of Takata and Chujiro Hayashi, things were as separated as they are today.

- Level one was taught into four main parts with four attunements.
- Level two had two main attunements.
- Level three had two attunements.

There are several Reiki schools, and each will have its way of passing these attunement levels. Some like to stick to the traditional way. Others like to take a modern approach. You could get several attunements for every degree, or they will just have one attunement for two or three levels of Reiki at once. It will all depend on the teacher and how they choose to pass their Reiki students.

It doesn't matter how it is done. The attunements are all reached because it happens through universal energy.

Reiki Levels

As we know them today, we have three Reiki levels:

- Shoden – beginner
- Okuden – inner hidden
- Shinpiden – mystery

Reiki Level 1 - Shoden

Reiki level one is shoden, or the beginner teachings. This is the level where you learn about the main principles, which is one of the pillars of Reiki.

- You learn hands-on techniques, how you can work with yourself, and how to perform self-treatments.
- The 21 days, a very important concept of Reiki
- How to communicate with your spirit guides

At this level, you start to learn how you can work with yourself. You will know more about the various vibration stages through which your energetic, physical, and emotional body. It is a more metaphorical beginner's level. This is because you start out getting to know yourself better through meditation and practicing on yourself.

This is where you will learn that you are a channel or instrument through which universal energy flows and manifests itself. Reiki will place your spiritual, emotional, mental, and physical body in a state of healing. As universal energy moves through you, it helps to cleanse your energy and blockages. This can help clear out depression, fears, and anxiety, and will help you reach a higher level of consciousness and awareness. This awareness will grow as you learn to focus on yourself. You will learn how to spot what needs to be balanced and healed. With time, you will start to learn how to understand others and the world around you.

The Reiki Principles are:

- "Just for today, I will be grateful."
- "Just for today, I will not anger."
- "Just for today, I will not worry."
- "Just for today, I will do my work honestly."
- "Just for today, I will respect all life."

These should be recited each morning, each night, and whenever you do Reiki or feel like you need to say them. Everything comes from within.

As mentioned, on the first level, you will learn the hands-on method of healing. Through activating your hands, you will learn how to place them in the correct positions. This enables you to channel energy and helps you to remove negative and residual energy.

Once you can do this, you can free yourself from energetic and mental blockages.

The purpose of these positions is to help heal the primary energy centers within the body and help create a strong flow that you will grow more aware of. It is best if you start from the head and move down so that all unwanted energy will flow down the body and then into the ground.

21 Day Self-Treatment

As soon as you start learning Reiki, you should perform the 21 days of self-treatment. It doesn't matter what time you do this. The important thing is to make sure you set aside the time for silence and peace to do the self-treatment.

People will typically fall into one of these three categories:

- Extra sensitive – people who feel even the slightest change in their energy and can tell you about it in great detail
- Normal sensitive – people who can feel the energy flow but don't feel the small changes
- Insensitive – people who have a hard time feeling and describing their energy flow

No matter where you live on that spectrum, Reiki works, and the energy is flowing. With regular practice, it won't matter if you are extra-, normal-, or insensitive. This is because you start in balance and feel the natural flow of energy. During these 21 days, it is the best time for you to calibrate yourself to new vibrations and universal energy.

These 21 days are meant to symbolize the 21 days Mikao Usui spends meditation and fasting. This is considered a "healing crisis," and while it can be a bit rough, it got its name from the changes in your body on an energetic level.

During this time, people can experience crying and yawning, while others feel hyper-energized or exhausted. Others may go through slightly more rough symptoms like dizziness or nausea. Don't worry. All of these things are normal, and they will stop once you become more balanced. Reiki helps your body to detoxify at an emotional, physical, and mental level.

It is recommended, but not required that you avoid meat-based meals or consuming large amounts of alcohol. You do need to make sure you drink plenty of water to flush out your toxins. If you are on medication, you should continue to do so.

Reiki is meant to help us grow and heal, but we also live in a physical world, so modern medicine does have its use. While many doctors are skeptical about alternative methods of healing, the two can still work together. During these 21 days, it is a time for healing inside and out. It is a time to get to know yourself and understand what you need to change for your greater good.

The last thing in level one is spirit guides. One of the most important things that you will learn within Reiki is how to work with your spirit guides. These are all positive, energetic entities from other planes of existence. We all have at least one spirit guide, but we often don't know how to communicate with it.

As you receive your Reiki attunements, you will also receive spirit guides. These spirit guides can help enhance your power during self-treatment and when you treat others. It can also help you out in your daily life.

Reiki Level 2 – Okuden

Once you reach this level, it is all about hidden inner teachings. The first degree was all about working with yourself from a physical perspective, and this level focuses more on the emotional and mental aspects. What does this mean?

Once you are attuned to this level, you will have access to a higher vibration, a healthy energy flow, and better awareness of your actual emotional and mental condition. This is when you will become more aware of your ability to channel energy through your emotional body, time, and space.

There is a crucial aspect of this level. The more you practice, the more you will bring to light the root of your imbalances. This is because you become more aware of them and will slowly start to heal from the source. This will help you have a clean, well built emotional and mental foundation.

These things will come to the surface and heal when they are meant to. It will all depend on you to start working with yourself first. With more experience, you will begin to learn how to do the same for other people. When you are at this level, you will discover that there isn't space, past, or future, but only the present. This level consists of:

- Becoming more aware and reaching a higher vibration that comes with the attunement to this level
- Learning the sacred Reiki symbols
- The power, mental-emotional, distance, and two non-traditional symbols that can help you heal your heart and communication

You will also learn how you can use those symbols to help cleanse and energize yourself, and others.

Reiki Level 3 – Shinpiden

This is also known as the mystery teachings. Many Reiki schools see this as a master's degree. This level is made up of:

- An improved ability to channel universal energy
- Learning more about what a Reiki Master is and what they are responsible for
- The master symbol, as well as information about what it brings

A Reiki practitioner will have to undergo some serious spiritual awakening before they reach level three. Some teachers decide that they don't want to pass this attunement onto others, but they still want to deepen their knowledge about Reiki. Therefore, it is often split into two attunements.

- The first is for the third degree and provides you with all of the knowledge, but you don't get the chance and information to share attunements with others.
- The other gives you the information to pass on attunements and knowledge for the third level.

This level is just the start of a potential spiritual evolution that lives within you. It is all up to you to bring this to the surface.

Energetic Systems

We know that Reiki is a set group of Japanese practices that come together to make a system that supports spiritual healing and growth. But what are the energetic systems that these principles are based on? Since Reiki was started in the early 1900s, we know that the tanden or hara were considered to be the middle of our energy powerhouse.

Hara translates to belly, stomach, or abdomen. Energy is stored within this area of the body and will then expand throughout the rest of the body. The teachings of Usui Mikao focuses on building up the energy in the hara. From the notes of Takata's diary, we have learned that she was taught to practice this way as well. After Reiki became westernized in the 1980s, they introduced the chakra system and replaced the old system.

The hara system is still one of the primary focuses for building energy within traditional teachings and exercises. There are two energy centers within the body, according to the Japanese energetic system. One of them is the head, and the other one is the heart. These are known as the Three Diamonds. By making a point of linking all their areas, the practitioner helps to form balance and unity. However, the most important thing is to develop a lower hara, as this is the central axis.

Through reestablishing a connection between energy and the hara, you can ensure good health and improved illness recovery. There will always be access to a reliable source of strength when needed. A person's inner attitude comes from focusing on the hara. From that point, people can find the ability to cope with their daily tasks and sudden emergencies with ease and understanding. This provides them with the ability to take appropriate action that is balanced and unbiased.

1. Earth Energy – Hara

This energy is located around three inches below the belly button, which would be in the sacral chakra area. This is where the original energy is stored. This is your life energy, and we are all born with this energy. This is your essence and provides you with purpose. At conception, you received your original energy from your parents, and this is the most important energetic connection you have with the universe. When hara, in a singular sense, is mentioned, it is this hara that is being discussed.

2. Heavenly Energy

This energy is connected to your spirit. When you become connected to this energy center, you could notice colors or a psychic ability you have never had before. You mustn't become unbalanced, so make sure you stay centered. If this energy can be used in a balanced way, you can see past the immediate moment.

3. Heart Energy

This energy is the center of your emotions. This is human energy that helps you to connect with the human experience. Through this area, you will learn what your life's purpose is. This journey will take you from your childhood to your adulthood and the return to being a child. As a child, you didn't have any experiences, but as you grew older, you become a child that has had experiences. This gives you a different point of view about life.

These three diamonds of energy are at the foundation of Reiki. They also play a big part in other aspects of Japanese culture, philosophy, and religion.

Usui Shiki Ryoho

One of the most common Reiki healing systems is the Usui system. Phyllis Lei Furumoto, a lineage bearer, defined Usui Shiki Ryoho as having four aspects: mystic order, spiritual discipline, personal development, and healing practice. Combining these things and the way they work together creates a system that has been found to help take people along a profound path of spiritual deepening, healing, and growth. If there are areas that end up getting changed or omitted, this form isn't recognized and becomes a new type of Reiki practice.

The more profound meaning and importance of all of these aspects and elements within the system is beyond words and will only unfold as you experience it. Here are some of the basics that you can expect from this system.

- Four Aspects
    - Healing Practice – Usui Shiki Ryoho is based on self-treatment and a type of treatment that can be used to treat other people. This can be reached through a series of treatment hand positions.
    - Personal Development – Through practicing this system, students will be presented with everyday choices. The choices will address their underlying beliefs and principles that they have acquired during their life. These beliefs and guides tend to be challenged as they might not be helpful for the person.
    - Spiritual Discipline – One of the inherent parts of practice is the connection to the spirit within each of us. This connection can cause the students to consider this as a spiritual practice.
    - Mystic Order – The practice of Usui Shiki Ryoho provides you with a sense of purpose and connection.

- Nine Elements
    - Oral Tradition – This system gets passed along through a person to person

relationship with a master through verbal and non-verbal communication, as well as energetic transmissions.

o Spiritual Lineage – The spiritual lineage of Reiki is made up of Phylis Lei Furumoto, Hawayo Takat, Chujiro Hayashi, and Mikao Usui. These lineage bearers embody the essence of this system. The teachings will be passed along the lines of masters, developing with their experiences, cultural norms of their times, and development of society.

o History – The story told between the teacher and the student gets passed through oral tradition during their first level classes. This is typically the story of Reiki. History doesn't typically focus on the actual people, but how Reiki has been passed down through the various lineage bearers.

o Initiation – The sacred and secret ritual gets passed along the lineage to the masters of this system. The masters will then connect their students to the energy of Reiki.

o Symbols – The three symbols that second level practitioners learn are accompanied by certain types of practices. The symbols act as energetic keys that can help a person connect with the non-physical world. This helps to prepare students for more significant choices in life and having a better understanding of the world.

o Treatment – This consists of various hand positions that a person holds for a few minutes in a specific order. This is the formal treatment process of Reiki. The informal treatment is made up of any hand position practiced with the other person's consent for as long as needed.

o   Form of Teaching – The form is where the teaching takes place for first and second level classes.

o   Monetary Exchange – Each initiatory step will require a certain amount of monetary commitment from the student.

o   Precepts – The five precepts are used to help awaken questions within the student. They require the student to use their mind body and spirit so they can become a whole body and spirit once again.

This is the most common practice Reiki system, as it is the original system. However, if you choose to take a different path to become a Reiki practitioner, that is okay as well. Universal energy is the same, no matter how you choose to access it.

Chapter 6:
Cleansing The Aura

When a person mentions an aura, they refer to the unseen spiritual energy field that surrounds every living thing. Everything alive will have an aura. The aura can be of various colors, and this can provide you with valuable insight into your spiritual and emotional wellbeing. While we might not be able to see them with the naked eye, we do have the power to feel auras. Think about the last new person you met. Did you notice if they have a friendly vibe, gave off negative energy, or felt warm? You can draw these conclusions before they ever say a word because you are reading their aura.

There are seven auric layers to your aura. They are also sometimes called planes or bodies, and each layer represents a different thing. You can even look at them like layers of an onion, with the middle of it being your physical body.

The first layer is the physical aura plane. This layer is what represents your physical health. This layer is the closest to your skin and is also called the etheric plane.

The second layer is the emotional aura plane. This layer corresponds to your emotions. If you are feeling rather emotional, then this plane is going to stand out. The aura can change colors depending on the mood of the person, and it can appear smudged or dull if they are experiencing emotional turmoil.

The third layer is the mental aura plane. This plane deals with thoughts, logic, and reasoning.

The fourth layer is the astral body aura plane. This layer is what deals with spiritual health. This is also the area in which you store your capacity for love.

The fifth layer is the etheric aura plane. This layer is where your psychic abilities lie. When the etheric plane is clear, it is easier for you to tap into the energy of others and connect with those who have matching wavelengths.

The sixth layer is the celestial aura plane. This is the layer that stores your intuition and dreams. This is also where your enlightenment lies. Someone who has a strong celestial aura plane will also be very creative.

The seventh layer is the causal aura plane. This helps to harmonize all of the other layers, and it is your guiding light on your life path.

Aura Colors

We also know that the aura has different colors, and they correspond with the seven main chakras. The aura also has a connection with those chakras. When you see what the colors correspond with, it can help you to interpret what your aura is trying to let you know.

Red is the color of your root chakra. When your aura contains red, it lets you know that you are working from a stable base.

Orange is the color of the sacral chakra. When your aura contains orange, and it lets you know that you are the emotional equivalent of resting under your weighted blanket. It means that you are a realist and independent.

Yellow is the color of the solar plexus chakra. When this color shows up in your aura, it means that you are optimistic, creative, and curious.

Green and pink relate to your heart chakra. When one of these colors appear in your aura, it often means that you are loving, compassionate, and kind.

Blue is connected to your throat chakra. When blue appears in your aura, it means that you are empathetic and intuitive.

Violet and purple relate to your third eye chakra. When these colors show up in your aura, it could indicate that you have some type of psychic ability and that you are extremely intuitive.

White is connected to the crown chakra, and having a white aura is extremely rare. This is what connects you to "All That Is" and provides you with the understanding that everybody is connected.

Black can show up in the aura, and it lets you know that you are holding onto something negative. That means you don't have a free-flow of energy.

Aura Cleansing

There are different methods to see what your aura is- one of the most common being aura photography. If you live in a big city, there is a good chance that there is somebody around that can read your aura. There is a chance that you may catch a glimpse of your aura. You may notice it as you walk past a mirror, or through meditation However, you don't have to see your aura to know whether or not you need to cleanse your aura.

You could just feel a bit off. Maybe you spill your coffee, drop a plate, get flipped off, hurt a person's feelings, and struggle with the essential things you should do at work. Then you may end up getting an unexpected bill, a friend reveals a long-buried grievance with you, you have to flake on an important meeting, and your car battery is dead when you try to go home.

These occurrences can seem relatively rare, but they are often less rare than we'd all like. Take a moment to think about those times, and how you have to figure out how to pull your energy out of the gutter.

This is how you can know when your aura needs to be cleansed.

Reiki masters worldwide will tell you that your aura is in a constant flux state due to the ever-changing world and emotions we experience. It can also affect the "vibe" that you give off. After that type of day, you will likely have some negative vibes because you won't feel all that great.

The thing is, you don't have to have a day like that to cause your aura to need to be cleaned. Sometimes, the signs you need to clean your aura can all be in your head and thoughts. Anytime you start feeling down on yourself, depressed, anxious, easily annoyed, or anything of that nature, this tells you that your aura needs cleansing. This "bubble" of energy that we all live in is ours to keep intact, clean, and free. You are responsible for your aura, and if you don't take care of it, you could be spreading negativity without knowing it. With that, let's look at some ways to cleanse your aura.

Running Energy

The first is running energy. Just like how our body benefits from regular exercise, running energy helps our spiritual practice. You can do this every day, but start with small doses. You should only take about five or ten minutes each day to ground yourself, run the energy, and then clear out the energy twice a day. As you get used to this practice, and you start to notice the benefits of more focus, vitality, and clarity, you may choose to increase the time you spend doing this. The great thing about this practice is that you don't have to have a tranquil space or a quiet room. You can do this in the store, during a meeting, or even during an argument.

While you may not be using hand placements and symbols, you are still working with Reiki energy. When you first do this, you may not feel anything, and that's fine. The important thing is that you continue doing it. Ask for the energy to come in, and trust that it is work within you. Continuing to practice this will help you progress towards your goals.

The first thing you have to do is get yourself grounded. We rarely live in the present. The stressors and activities in our daily life cause us to find ourselves ruminating about the past or worrying about the future. Getting grounded means you bring yourself into the present. This presence gives you a doorway into healing and is the most essential thing you can do when you start this process.

1. Create your ground cord from your root chakra.

Start by sitting upright with your feet flat on the floor and your arms uncrossed. You want your body to be as straight as possible to allow for the free-flow of energy. Picture a beam of light or a cord traveling out of the root chakra down into the earth below you, grounding you.

2. Allow your seventh chakra to open.

Next, you will need to picture a beam of light coming out of your crown chakra and moving straight up into the sky, connecting you with cosmic energy.

3.   Call your spirit home.

Next, you are going to have to say your complete name out loud three times. The reason you do this is that your name is unique to only. When this is done, it helps to pull you into the present moment.

4.   Create more grounding cords from your feet.

You now need to wake up the energy in your feet. With your feet planted on the floor, imagine that a beam of light is moving from the middle of your feet down into the earth.

5.   Run with the earth's energy.

Once you have all of the cords established, along with the cosmic energy moving through the crown chakra, you can start to pull up the earth's energy. This energy is forest green. Ask the earth to release energy up through your feet, legs, torso, and then out of the crown. Allow this to move through you until it has filled all of the outer layers of your body until it reaches the edges of your aura. Once you feel that your body and aura have been filled with this forest green earth energy, let the energy flush out of you and back into the earth.

6.   Run with forgiveness.

Imagine that this energy is translucent gold with just a bit of a blue hue to it. Like you did before with the earth energy, you will want to pull the energy up through the soles of your feet, up the legs, and through the body. Allow this energy to flow out of your crown and fill up your aura. As this energy moves through your aura, it will push away any energy that is not serving your best interest, making more room for your spirit. Once you feel your body and aura is filled with the energy, release it back down through your feet and into the earth. You should make sure that you repeat this four times.

You are now entirely grounded, and your body and mind are ready for the next part.

Once you have grounded yourself, you will be able to pull energy through your chakras more easily. This will help to cleanse them by getting rid of blockages. You are going to understand better what your body needs.

7. Run with cosmic energies.

The grounding energies you worked with earlier came up through the earth and fill you and your aura before flushing back into the ground along with the ground cords. However, the cosmic energies we are going to use now will travel through your crown and move down the chakras. They will travel down your grounding cord and will stop moving once they reach the earth. It is best if you run the following energies four times each, and make sure that you imagine all of the colors moving throughout your body as you do this.

First is deprogramming energy. This should be imagined as a deep royal blue, and it will help to wash out any dense vibrational energy that you may have.

The second is the clarity of energy. This is a neon-electric blue color that will help to enhance your clarity and expand your knowingness.

The third is the healing energy. This is a green color that helps to heal wounds.

Fourth is the love and truth energy. The color of this one is golden, and it helps to revitalize you with light and reminds you of who you are.

8.   Replacing your ground cord and bringing the practice to a close.

This is probably one of the most essential parts of this process. You need to make sure that you replace your grounding cords with new ones, which will help to anchor you into your present moment. Allow all of the residual energy to move through you and release it down your current cord. Then, the old cord will be removed by picturing a rose rooted deep within the earth. The rose you are picturing symbolizes forgiveness, and it helps to transmute any dense energy that is leftover into the light. Let that old cord be moved into the center of the rose and watch it explode into pieces over the ocean. Watch as it is washed away to be renewed. Then you will repeat steps one through four. After that, you will be ready to move on with your day, living in the present and complete harmony.

Cleansing Bath or Shower

There is a very good reason why you always leave a shower or bath feeling refreshed and inspired. You can also cleanse your aura by taking an aura cleansing bath, and this is a great thing to do after any Reiki healing sessions.

This is a ritualistic process where you will use salts, sacred herbs, and essential oils to help clean your energy field. All you will need to do is fill up your bathtub, and then add in a few drops of lavender or eucalyptus essential oil and add in a cup of Epsom or Himalayan sea salt. You can also choose to add in some rose or sandalwood essential oils to help up the cleansing effect of the bath.

You will need to soak in this bath for at least ten minutes. However, if you don't have time for a bath and would prefer to take a shower, picture your aura being healed and repaired as the water travels down your body. Imagine that all negativity is moving out of your body as the water drains out of the tub.

You should also make sure that you picture divine energy moving throughout your body as you wash, and picture that you are surrounded by a white light bubble. Once your bath is over, make sure that you discard any herbs or flowers that you may have used.

Dance In The Rain

This is a fun and easy way to cleanse your aura. You don't have to wait to do this one when you are feeling negative or drained. Whenever you have a nice rain, you can do this. Make sure it is only raining and is not a storm. All you have to do is go outside and walk around in the rain. As you do this, allow the raindrops to soak you thoroughly. Imagine that all of the toxicity and negativity getting washed out of you by the rain. You can get a similar effect by going for a swim in a lake. Again, you should not do this if the rain is accompanied by thunder and lightning.

Aura Combing

Before you do an aura combing, make sure that you thoroughly wash and dry your hands. You will want to find a quiet and comfortable place in your home to do this. Start by visualizing your aura, and then close your eyes. Start to use your hands to comb through the space around you. You will want to start at the top of your head and comb the area around you, moving down to your toes. You must visualize your aura being cleansed each time that you comb through your space. Once you feel as though your aura is cleansed, you will want to end the session by thoroughly washing your hands once more to get rid of the negative energy.

Chapter 7:
Cleansing Yourself

I looked into Reiki after I was diagnosed with adrenal fatigue and autoimmune disease. I could not deny the role that stress played in my life, and on the journey to get my stress under control, several other symptoms popped up their ugly heads, then I found Reiki. It gave me a tangible practice that helped me relieve pains and aches, process all those hard emotions while staying resilient in the middle of life's challenges.

Some of these challenges were a full-time job and constant burnout. Just the thoughts of commuting, working, going home, and not having any energy for the rest of my life filled me with dread. But I wanted to keep my independence and my career was important. The job I had, had very little importance, but it was still a part of my career path. Things had to change, but it couldn't be my lifestyle or job.

All I wanted was more energy. I wanted a way to get it that was more than detoxing or dieting. I have always been an empathy, and my burnout was a lot deeper than being physical. Once I found Reiki, I had found a tool that helped me feel more empowered. I could take energy into my own hands wherever and whenever I needed it.

Even though Reiki is never meant to take the place of scientifically-backed strategies, it could be used to complement other healing practices. Although you can't do Reiki on yourself until you have completed level one training, you can use some healing techniques to help you during this quarantine and later in life. As with any tool used to transform, growth will when you continuously show up and practice. This means that you need to commit to doing this regularly.

Meet Reiki

Reiki comes from "Rei," a Japanese word that means universal life, and the word "Ki," which means energy. So, simply put, Reiki means universal life force energy. If you are living, you have this energy, and you have everything you need to heal yourself.

Try this exercise: Put your hands together and rub them briskly for a couple of seconds. Now just hold them there. Slowly move them away from each other until they are a couple of inches apart. You should feel some sensations like a buzzing between your hands. Now place your hands over your eyes and notice the warm feeling. This is your life force. This is your superpower. Practicing Reiki could help you build a relationship and get to know your power.

This is a very subtle power. It is a lot quieter than wind or a jolt of caffeine. In my experience, when you tune into that energy, it is usually all the medicine you need when you are feeling depleted.

My Philosophy

Reiki, to me, is an energetic dialogue that I have with myself. This is when I unite my mind and body with an intention that I ask myself: "Okay, where am I at today? What is happening to this body?" This is where I step into the healer role and give myself some love. Anything that lets us accept and feel our emotional and energetic state could be potent and healing. I don't have to know "if Reiki works." I already know that it works great for me, and I think anyone who is curious needs to try it.

Body Scan Ritual That Can Connect You To Your Energy

Lie down on a yoga mat or blanket. Just make sure you are comfortable. Set a timer for the amount of time you have.

Dry bathe your body by brushing your arms down to your hands and then toward the floor. Now do this with the insides of your arms. Do this three or four times. Don't use a regular hairbrush. You need to get a body brush.

Bring your hands up to your heart while setting an intention for your Reiki. It could be something simple like: "I want to feel grounded in my body."

Now visualize a white beam of healing light flowing into your crown chakra and going down through your entire body. It will be spreading healing energy while it travels.

Put your hand on top of your head and move them slowly down over your whole body. You aren't touching your body here, just hovering a few inches above your body. You need to follow your hand with your breath and remember to breathe into every body part when you move over it.

If you find that any of these spaces feel heavy or icky, take a few minutes to work on these areas to cleanse out the excess energy. You will need to use your intuition while you are doing this.

Once you are done, "sweep" the energy away from the body and get rid of it. Bring your hands back to your heart in gratitude.

Ways You Can Practice Healing Yourself with Reiki Consistently

Support Your Body

Start your practice by finding a posture that is comfortable but supports your mind and body while relaxing. I will either lie down or sit on a meditation cushion cross-legged. If you decide to sit cross-legged, make sure that your hips are above your knees for the best comfort. If you lie down, support your neck and knees with some cushions. You could also sit in a chair with your feet firmly on the ground. This helps you stay grounded. You might have to experiment until you have found a posture that is restful but engaging.

Honor Intentions

The best thing you can do to stick with your choices is to show up and practice. You have already set the time, remembered it was time to practice, and gotten the courage to practice. Sitting down with your loud emotions, uncomfortable sensations, and racing mind is a bit intimidating. Just know that every day you show up with some compassion, it is a day to celebrate.

Meditate

Now, draw your attention inward and focus on your breathing. See if you can find any areas in your body that feel achy or tense. Send your breath and awareness to that point. Drop your shoulders down and open your heart's center. Relax the muscles in your face and make sure you aren't clenching your teeth. Continue scanning your body to find any other points and send your breath and awareness there until you feel entirely embodied.

Now, send your breath into your lower belly. When you breathe into this part of the body, it anchors your mind and vibrates the vagus nerve. This can cultivate your vitality while centering and grounding you in the present moment.

Precepts

Mikao Usui gave us the five precepts when he shared this practice with his students in 1922. This is the framework for living your life to the fullest.

During your self-healing practice, you can recite the precepts several times as a way to practice your emotional and mental hygiene. You could discover that your goals in life, relationships, health, and spiritual evolution are led by the following five precepts:

- Today only

- Don't anger

- Don't worry

- Be grateful

- Practice diligently

- Show compassion to others and yourself

Call Your Guides

This is an optional step, but you can welcome your spirit guides. Place your hand in a prayer pose and repeat a simple prayer like: "I welcome the presence of my Reiki masters, guides, healers, and teachers. I welcome all your energetic blessings and messages for the highest good of all. Thank you for gracing us with your light and love." Let their presence be heard, felt, or seen, and it doesn't matter how dramatic or subtle it might be.

Use Hands-On Healing

Even though you have to receive attunements by a Reiki master to channel Reiki, anybody can channel light and love by using the power of their spirit guides, breath, awareness, and intentions. Everybody possesses Reiki, and they use it every day without even realizing it. When your child falls and scrapes their knee, you will automatically put your hand on their knee and rub it. You are unconsciously working with life force energy. You are channeling and sending energy, and the child is drawing in and receiving that energy.

You might start practicing hands-on healing without having an attunement. If you are interested in channeling and sensing Reiki energy, it would be best to take a Reiki training class and have an attunement.

Give Thanks

Take some time to thank your guides, Reiki energy, and yourself for creating the process of self-healing by using Reiki. Thank the journey that got you to Reiki. Trust in the life force that has balanced your soul, body, mind to its highest alignment while gently releasing the bad energy.

Reiki energy is always inside you and is always available to be used. Even if you haven't been trained in Reiki, you can still do some self-healing. By getting into a comfortable position, meditating, saying the precepts, you can start your self-healing journey. It just takes some willingness and courage to show up for this revolution.

Give Yourself a Reiki Bath

Being in quarantine has made many people turn to spirituality to try and make sense of this world. Most people have their shaman, clergy, pastor, etc., on speed dial, while others are looking to Instagram for breathing gurus. If you feel like your need a complete overhaul, it might be time to take a Reiki bath.

Reiki can be used to get rid of stagnancies and blockages that are impeding the flow of energy within our bodies to promote our emotional and physical well being.

Jasmin Harsono, a Reiki master, wrote a book about the best way to heal yourself with Reiki. The book features some practices and rituals that can help with things like relieving anxiety to getting more sleep.

Her book, *Self Reiki*, breaks down the five elements that make up the components of Reiki.

People who are new to Reiki should only worry about the first three. These components are: the principles of Reiki, a practice code that helps you live mindfully and positively, meditation and mindfulness techniques that can deepen your connection, and healing hands is a method of using your palms to share "ki" to offer to heal to others and ourselves.

Touch is a powerful sensation, and it is as ancient as humans. Anytime we get hurt, we will automatically rub or cover the area that got damaged. If another person is in pain, we will offer them comfort. Our hands are where most people feel their connection with life force energy. Once you have connected to Reiki, your hands might begin to tingle, get warmer, or feel lighter or heavier. You can use your hands to share "ki" with others.

If you want to take Reiki to the next level and want to do Reiki healing on others, the next stage will be to have some attunements. This is when a Reiki master will share their universal energy with you.

Here are some simple beginner techniques you can practice:

Make A Sanctuary

Create a space inside your home that is dedicated just to your meditation. This sanctuary needs to be prepared for you whenever you need it. This sanctuary will be ready for you when you enter it each day.

Do A Grounding Meditation

Anytime you are feeling unbalanced, you need to ground yourself so that you feel rooted. This would be an excellent exercise to do after a deep meditation as it helps you come "back to earth" when you have tuned into your psychic ability or intuition. Take some time to let your connection to earth fully develop.

Every morning, begin your day with a five to ten-minute meditation to ground yourself. Build a practice of breathing into your gut. This practice can help ground your physical body to help you feel clear and centered. Space will be created in your belly so you can begin experiencing Reiki that will support your spirit, body, and mind.

Inhale deeply into your belly and say: "breathing in." When you exhale, push out all the stagnant energy while saying: "Breathing out."

Imagine yourself rooted firmly in the ground, with a cord that goes from your belly deep into the earth under you. Sense this grounding in your soul, mind, and body.

Feel connected and grounded at the moment, just like you are. Inhale again and exhale completely. Put your hands in a "prayer pose" and open your eyes.

Indulge in a Full Treatment

Having a full body treatment each day will help deepen your experience with Reiki. You will begin feeling and understanding what your mind and body need at every moment.

After performing the meditation, rest your hands over each of your chakras for a few minutes, starting at the crown, and then moving down to the root chakra.

A Reiki bath will use the same hand positions as a full treatment, with the sensory experience being heightened by lying in a warm bath and listening to some soothing music. You can light candles or place some crystals in your bath water, as long as they are not water-soluble crystals. If you decide to use crystals make sure you research to find out if they can be safely used in water. Some can end up melting, and this can end up hurting you. We want to heal. Not cause more problems.

Journal Your Practice

This is going to help expand on what happens to you during your meditation. It can help you understand your feelings, thoughts, and sensory experiences that might come up. Every day you will be able to see how you have advanced and how it is helping you.

Practice the Precepts

To incorporate the Reiki precepts into your life and meditation, you have to chant or say them daily. You can easily say:

"Just for today. Don't worry. Don't be angry. Be grateful. Work with diligence and be kind to yourself and other people."

These principles are the essence of what Reiki is. You need to learn how to release the past and the future and live solely in the moment. Focus on your higher vibrations of kindness and gratitude to support your life. This helps you to share more positivity and spread happiness to the world.

Gassho Meditation

This might look like a lot of steps, this is a very simple meditation, and after you have mastered it, you will find that it has become second nature.

First Step

Make sure that you are sitting comfortably. The spine should be straight, but make sure that you are also comfortable. Your head should be upright and in a neutral position.

You need to make sure you don't strain yourself to get into this position. If you have problems with your back, or it is hard for you to sit still, you can sit in a chair with a few pillows at your back.

You could sit on the floor on a cushion and press your back on the wall. You can also choose to get comfortable on the couch or bed, but you might fall asleep, which isn't going to do any good.

Second Step

Let your eyes close and press the palm of your hands together. Place your closed hands in front of your heart. Ensure that your thumbs are resting in the center of your chest, right where the heart chakra is located. When you release your breath through your nose, you should be able to feel your breath on your fingers.

Third Step

Focus on the area where your middle fingers are touching. Allow everything else to drop from your mind. If you notice that your mind wanders, acknowledge that thought and then release it. Focus on bringing your attention back to where your fingers are touching each other.

Do your best not to think about anything else. Watch these thoughts just like you would do if you were watching a movie. Just let those thoughts brush to the side. You always want to bring yourself back to where your fingers are touching. You want to make sure that your hands are relaxed. This means that you don't have a bunch of tension in your hands. Make sure that your hands are only touching and are not being pressed together.

Fourth Step

You could feel as though this position isn't comfortable to hold for 30 minutes. If your hands do start to hurt, then allow them to drop but keep them together. Now continue the meditation.

Fifth Step

You could notice that the energy appears to you in the form of images, cold, or heat.

It's fine if your notice them, but make sure that you let them go and come back to the point where your fingers are touching. Make sure you don't allow yourself to get caught up in these new sensations. If you feel as though you need to adjust your posture, then do this slowly and with conscious and deliberate movements.

Sixth Step

Make sure that your eyes are closed, and rest your hands on your lap while enjoying the peacefulness for just a couple of minutes. Make sure that you remind yourself that you hold a lot of peace within your heart at all times. It is always going to be there whenever you meditate.

Seventh Step

Take a couple of full, deep breaths and then start to focus on your eyes as you open them.

The majority of Reiki practitioners find that this type of mediation helps to bring them more clarity and focus in their daily lives, and it will help them to become more centered and relaxed. It also gives them more creativity and productivity in their day. You don't have to practice Reiki to practice this form of meditation.

Chapter 8:
Cleansing Others

It is imperative that you create an appropriate setting, if possible when you are doing a Reiki cleansing session. You can do it in your home if you have a spare room that you can use just for cleansing. If this isn't possible, you might want to check into joining a local healing center. If this is the case, you can rent a cleansing room at a reasonable price.

Whatever room you decide to use needs to be clean and light and makes others feel safe. Bright pastel colors, like purple, white, or yellow, can be used to help you reach the effect that you desire. You have to make sure that nothing will interrupt you. Make sure you disconnect or unplug your doorbell and phones. If you are working in your home, be sure to let your family members know that you will be working with a client, so they don't bother you.

If at all possible, use a therapy table. You could use a strong table and put some thick blankets on top to make it more comfortable. You are going to need two pillows. One will go under your client's head while the other goes under their feet. You need to make sure that the room is at a comfortable temperature. Some people tend to get cold when they lie still, so have some extra blankets handy that you can cover them with if needed.

Add some plants to your room to give it a homey feeling. You can also place some crystals under the table to help fix some of the energies. Some prefer to have the room completely silent when they are cleansing, but others like playing some Reiki music in the background. This will help your client relax. Music can also help you relax, and this lets you focus on cleansing. Nature sounds like water, dolphins, and whales can be relaxing, too.

You can find many CDs on the market that are made for Reiki treatment sessions. They are made so that they play for the entire length of the Reiki sessions that has a chime or bell sound added at three or five-minute intervals that let you know when you should move your hands.

Burning essential oils or incense could add a pleasing aroma to the room, too. But just be careful as some people might be sensitive to specific smells, and it could cause them to have an unpleasant session. To keep this from happening, ask them before you light any incense or oils. During the cleaning session, you might realize that your client is crying while they release any blocked problems. Try to keep a box of tissues available if this happens.

To put the finishing touches on your space, you might want to hang some pictures of Jesus, Buddha, Madam Takata, Dr. Hayashi, or Dr. Usui. It all depends on who you call upon when you do your invocation or prayer.

Take Off Your Jewelry

Reiki can move through any materials like metal, concrete, brick, and stone. But the rocks and metal that are used to make jewelry can attract specific kinds of negative energy. To ensure your Reiki energy is free from any type of energy disturbance, it is best to take off all jewelry like necklaces, chains, earrings, watches, and rings.

People who work with crystals or gemstones that are used in healing know that these materials could become full of negative energy. This is why they need to be cleaned regularly.

Take Off Any Clothing That is Too Tight

For Reiki to flow through you and your client freely, you must make sure that you aren't wearing tight-fitting clothing like shoes, ties, or belts. This makes you both feel more relaxed and comfortable. Reiki can travel through clothes, so you shouldn't need to take off any more clothing. You might realize that it is more comfortable for you when you wear clothes that fight you loosely when you are working with cleansing.

Stay Away From Alcoholic Beverages

Alcohol can dissipate energy. You should not consume alcohol in the 24 hours before your session or during your session.

Be Aware Of Your Hygiene

Make sure that you look fresh and clean and that you smell pleasant. Don't wear any cologne, aftershave, or perfumes that have a strong smell. If you have a habit of smoking, you need to brush your teeth well and make sure you rinse with mouthwash before the session. Try your best not to eat onions, garlic, or other foods that could end up causing your breath to smell.

Make sure that your hands are washed before each session using a neutral or lightly scented soap. Your hands are going to touch your client's skin and face, so your hygiene and your client's peace of mind for your hands need to be clean.

Saying The Invocation

You need to remember that being a Reiki healer, you aren't healing your clients. Your clients are cleansing themselves. You are working as the channel that helps move the energy from your hands and into their body to heal them. This invocation symbolizes that you are not claiming any of the power. You are simply using yourself as a conduit the universal power will flow through.

While you don't have to use this invocation to turn on your Reiki energy, it does help to disassociate yourself from your ego. It also helps to pay respect to the universe and the person that you are working with.

You need to make sure that your prayer is personal and connected to your own beliefs. You also need to ask permission before you start acting as a channel for Reiki healing. I have written down my invocation that might help you create a prayer that is suitable for you to use.

After your client has laid down on the table is relaxed and ready to receive Reiki, move to the top of the table next to the client's head. Allow your eyes to close, and then place your hands in a prayer pose in front of your heart chakra. If you have your client seated, put your hands on their shoulders during the invocation.

Personal Invocation

You need to take a few minutes before you begin a treatment to get yourself ready to work on channeling Reiki. This time is great for getting in touch with your guides, assistants, or mentors. It lets you have a moment of reflection so you can focus your thoughts on the healing you will be doing. It's important to start with the correct mental attitude. You should wish to pass on unconditional healing and love in the purest sense.

You could say something like: "I call upon Reiki, all the Angelic beings, the Universal Life Forces who have worked with Reiki especially my spirit guides,

Madam Takata, Dr. Hayashi, Dr. Usui, and all the other Reiki master past, present, and future to draw near me and help me with this cleansing session."

"I ask that the wisdom and power of Reiki let me become a channel for its unconditional healing and love on behalf of (use client's name here). Allow Reiki's infinite wisdom to go where it is needed, and may it be used for the greater good. May we all be empowered by our Divine love and blessings. Amen."

Harmonize and Cleanse The Clients Aura

Before you start cleansing your client, make sure that you run your hands just above your client, around six inches, from their head to their feet using a smooth and slow motion three times to help remove built-up energy. This helps to bring more harmony into their aura and helps to create a strong connection between you and the client. Make sure that you keep your focus on your hands. It's okay to use your intuition to spot any large pockets of blockages that you should focus on during the cleansing.

The Treatment

Before beginning a full body cleanse, there are a few things that you need to keep in mind.

- You should never perform a treatment on a person who has diabetes and is taking insulin injections, especially if they are not prepared to start checking their insulin daily and reduce how much they need

- Don't treat anybody with a pacemaker since Reiki can affect the rhythm.

Make sure you explain to your client who you are working with for the first time exactly what you will be doing and the reactions they might have. Stress that any reaction they have will be completely normal. They could experience some of these reactions, if not all of them. They also might not have any reactions at all. It doesn't make any difference. Reiki will go where it is needed.

Reactions that they might have:

- A sense that your hands are moving

- Pins and needles

- Flashes of memory

- Tummy rumbling

- Emotional responses

- Itchiness

- Falling asleep

- Involuntary movements

- Flashes of your past lives

- Colors

- Feeling cold

- Feeling hot

Sometimes your client might experience some extreme coldness where your hands are positioned but you might feel the heat.

If your client doesn't experience anything, just explain that Reiki energy works on subtle levels but it will have wonderful results that will be more noticeable in the weeks and days after the treatment.

Don't forget your client is getting their Reiki energy from you. They are the ones that are healing on a subconscious level. You are simply being their channel.

Reiki Will Travel Where It Is Needed

You don't need to know anything about physiology or human anatomy to work with Reiki. Make sure that you leave your ego at home and make sure that you allow the Reiki to do its work.

Don't Worry About the Symptoms and Treat the Entire Person

You have to listen carefully to your client's body with your hands. Try your best to sense all the various energies. If the energy you are feeling is very strong, make sure that you keep your hands placed in the same position until you start to notice a change within the energy. You have to use your intuition. Try to see any non-verbal communications from their body. Leg or hand movements and sighing deeply are all good indications that something is happening.

The normal time that it will take for a complete body treatment is between one hour and 90 minutes.

Once the treatment is over, give your client some water to help them ground back into the moment. Remember to wash your hands again.

Starting the Treatment

Make sure the person is flat on the table and that their arms are laying next to their side. Their legs have to be flat against the table. Make sure they aren't crossed as this can block the Reiki energy from flowing.

Gently place your hands along their body. The hands should be kept in each position for about three to five minutes. The more experienced you become, the more you will be able to use your intuition.

You need to cup your hands and keep your fingers closed like you are trying to hold water in your hands. This will keep the channel strong between the Universal life force and your client. If the fingers open, Reiki energy could escape just like water will slip through open fingers.

When you get to your client's genital areas or breasts, don't touch them, just hover your hands above their body. If they have an area of burned skin, hover above this area, too.

Once all the positions have been treated, put your left hand over their crown chakra and your right hand at the bottom of their spine. This last position will balance the energy flowing through their body.

Finish the treatment by combing their aura. Stroke their body firmly from the crown chakra down to their feet in a sweeping motion. Go past their feet until you have touched the floor. This will help ground them and you. Repeat this with a lighter touch. And do it one more time with your hand about two inches above their body.

Quick Treatment

There might be sometimes when you realize that it won't be practical to take an entire hour or hour and a half doing a full Reiki treatment. They might be many reasons why a person only has a few minutes or you are needed by a family member in another room or place.

There is another quick version that could be used for this situation. The "Rapid Reiki Treatment" will focus on all of the chakras as the client is sitting upright in a chair. This will take between 15 and 30 minutes to do.

- First Position

Your client needs to be sitting in a chair. You will stand behind them. Put your hands on their shoulders. Silently say your invocation.

- Second Position

Stay behind your client. Put both of your hands on top of your head. Make sure you are covering their crown chakra.

- Third Position

Move around so that you are standing beside your client. Put one of your hands on their forehead over their third eye. Place the other hand over their occipital ridge located on the back of the head.

- Fourth Position

Stay beside your client and put one hand over their throat chakra at the middle of their neck and the other hand should be at the same place on the back of their neck. It will look as if you are trying to choke them.

- Fifth Position

Stay beside your client and put one hand over their heart charka in the middle of their chest. Put your other hand in between their shoulder blades.

- Sixth Position

Stay beside your client and put one hand over their solar plexus. Your other hand will be at their spine but make sure you keep it equal to the hand in front.

- Seventh Position

Stay beside your client and put one hand over the base of their stomach over their sacral chakra. Put your other hand on the base of their spine.

- Eighth Position

Move until you are in front of them and put one of your hands on each of their knees.

- Ninth Position

Kneel in front of them and put one hand over each of their feet. Move your thumbs out but keep your hands cupped over their feet on the floor.

Last but not least, comb their aura three times just like you would do at the end of a normal session. Take time to wash your hands in some cold water and provide them with a glass of water to help them ground back into the present.

If you don't feel comfortable doing the third through eight positions, you can sit in a chair beside them. Take between three and five minutes if your intuition doesn't tell you any different.

Ultradian Technique

Research has found that how bodies function in different cycles. One of these so-called cycles is the ultradian rhythm. This is the body's natural cycle of rest and activity. While we sleep, we will dream every 90 to 120 minutes. We will do this even if we don't remember the dream. During our normal daily lives, this rhythm will continue. In our normal daily activity, we might have a sudden urge to stop what we are doing and rest. Our body needs to take breaks every 90 to 120 minutes to maintain and repair itself.

Many people will misjudge this important and natural process and won't let themselves take this power break that they need. Rather than relaxing for a short time and recharging their batteries, they just give themselves a "power boost" by drinking a caffeinated drink like soda, tea, or coffee or by eating chocolate. These stimulants only cover their body's need for a break so it can maintain their well being and health. If we constantly ignore these breaks, we will upset the rhythms and balance of our spirit, body, and mind.

All of this neglect could lead to stress disorders and health problems like various psychological problems, eating disorders, sexual dysfunction, psychosomatic illnesses and pain, mood disorders, and stress disorders like depression. Reiki could be used to help prevent and treat this problem since it can bring the body back into normalizing the ultradian rhythm and equilibrium.

Throughout your day, try to notice any signs that your body might be giving you that is telling you to stop and rest. These signs might happen as a sudden feeling that you need to slow down or you have a sudden loss of energy. You might feel yourself drift into a trance-like state like you are daydreaming.

When this happens, take a short break and it will rejuvenate and revitalize your entire spirit, body, and mind. Put your cupped hands over your eyes. Close your eyes and go inside yourself.

Now, be aware of any part of your body that feels tired, sore, or tight. If you do find a part that needs Reiki healing, move your hand to that point and keep them there for as long you need. Try to visualize or sense that part being filled with Reiki energy.

Now, make that light grow larger and brighter until it encompasses your entire body. See if you can sense a feeling of well being and peace as this healing light fills your aura and create a protective shield of energy and love around you. Once you feel recharged and rejuvenated, slowly open your eyes and go about your day.

Repeat this regularly to keep your energy level high and to prevent illness and stress. It is very important to change the way you respond to your body's natural rhythms.

Get rid of eating junk food as a way to boost your energy by eating natural and healthier foods that will add years to your life.

If you don't find any parts of your body that needs Reiki healing, go internally once again and take another look. Sometimes it takes a second look to find which parts need to be healed. This happens because they are hidden deep in our unconscious minds. If you don't find anything just keep your hands over your eyes for as long as you have to. This break is still going to benefit your well being and health.

If conditions or time keeps you from taking a short break, there is another easy way to keep fighting against diseases and sickness. The thymus gland, found between your heart and throat chakra, is an organ that makes white blood cells that fight off infections. While it's not completely understood as to what the thymus's exact job is, it's understood that it plays an important role in creating immunities that help fight off diseases. This is done by making hormones that are essential for a person's immune system that is called the Thymic Humoral Factor.

Researchers think that this hormone acts with lymphocytes and makes them turn into a plasma that will form antibodies that create immunities.

You can gently tap between 20 and 30 times on your chest over your thymus gland or put one of your hands over this point for about three minutes. This technique will help you boost and maintain your immune system while filling your body with vital energy.

Reiki Group Treatment

Group treatments were often used by Dr. Hayashi. His clients were treated with the help of other Reiki healers. Many people find this to be enjoyable when working with others. There are some advantages when working as a group.

Benefits

Group treatments are quicker, and they only take about six to ten minutes to do an entire session. These kinds of treatments are extremely powerful. The client will receive a huge burst of energy that can heal them quickly. This usually causes the client's natural healing process to go into overdrive.

Group treatment lets a team create a bond, and this, in turn, will make some very unique energy. Since everyone experiences Reiki differently, clients might notice all the various vibrations that are coming from all the different practitioners.

How to Conduct Group Treatment

You will use all the same procedures and preparations of a normal Reiki treatment when doing group sessions. You have to decide who is going to work on the head as they will control the entire session before you ever begin a group session.

It all depends on the number of practitioners that you have in the group session as to which practitioner will be working with which hand position. Remember to figure out who is going to end the treatment by combing the aura.

If more than four practitioners are doing a treatment, you can place one practitioner at the client's head, one at their feet, and the other two will work in the center.

Group treatments are a great way to help many people if you don't have a lot of time. Make sure you take the time to wash your hands under cool water before a session and after a session to get rid of negative energy and to help ground you at the moment. Take some time and share your experiences. Group treatments are a great way to grow and learn with others. And don't forget the tissues.

Reiki Pregnancy, Babies, and Children

Pregnancy

Reiki is very beneficial and safe for a pregnant woman and her unborn baby. Women who have previously studied Reiki and have become in tune with the Universe and its life force have found their pregnancy to be enjoyable. Their childbirth was a lot easier and without complications. Reiki can help during pregnancy in the following ways:

- Helps with morning sickness

- Reduces tiredness and stress

- Stimulates the baby's development

- Helps treat pain in the spine, joints, or muscles

- Strengthens the connection between the baby and the mother. If the pregnant woman puts her hands against her stomach, she will be pushing love and healing to her child.

- Can keep your spirit, body, and mind balanced. It can reduce the chances of developing the "baby blues" or postpartum depression.

- Nourishes the fetus with love and the life force that comes from the Universe. It can gently envelop, protects, and comforts the baby

- The baby's daddy can help by giving the mother treatments if he is a Reiki practitioner. This will create a bond between the child and its father. It gets stimulated every time he puts his hands on the mother's belly. The father can communicate with his child through his hands

- Reiki can help a couple who is having a hard time conceiving a child by lessening their stress and stimulating the reproductive organs in both males and females. In most cases, if a couple is desperate for a child they are putting a lot of stress on themselves and this causes an imbalance in their spirit, body, and mind. When they finally give up and forget about having children, the stress and pressure go away and most couples find that they are pregnant soon afterward.

Babies

- Once the mother gives birth, Reiki can be used to speed up the recovery time for the newborn and the mother. This is very helpful with C-sections and healing all the stitches and scars that come with childbirth.

- Can help heal the baby's umbilical cord

- Nourishes and revitalizes mom's milk while breastfeeding

- The mom can treat the baby's formula with Reiki if she bottle feeds the baby.

- When the mother enriches and treats the baby's food, it could help satisfy and nourish the baby.

- Reiki can encourage the baby to feed until they are full and content.

- Full feedings can lead to the baby sleeping through the night faster. This is something that every parent looks forward to

- Stimulates the baby's balance. This gets channeled to the baby anytime the father or mother touches their child.

- Can help treat gassiness, colic, and cradle cap

Always talk to the baby's pediatrician anytime you get worried about your baby. It doesn't matter how trivial the problem might be.

Children

- Use it to treat your child during their entire lives.

- Use it during every stage of life like puberty, adolescence, and adulthood.

- Helps with all pains and aches such as those so-called "growing pains" that some children experience

- Most parents have an innate instinct to kiss or touch their children when they fall and get hurt.

- Can speed up healing while boosting the child's natural ability to heal themselves

- You can share this special gift with your child.

- Do your best to teach your child what the basic five principles are of Reiki and teach them to incorporate them in their lives.

- Children do enjoy Reiki, and if at all possible, you should introduce them to Reiki and help them attune themselves to it. It can help them find their path in life.

- Can help your child go to sleep better

- Balances your child's spirit, body, and mind. This can lead to a more focused and more straightforward approach to life at home and school.

- If a child has an accident, they usually cry due to the shock. You can treat your child by putting one hand over their solar plexus and the other hand over the base of their spine.

Conclusion

Thank you for making it through to the end of the book. Let's hope it was informative and able to provide you with all of the tools you need to achieve your goals, whatever they may be.

The next step is to start using what you have learned about Reiki and start healing yourself or others. It can help to practice personal healing techniques first, and once you feel like you have that under control, you can start offering to heal others. This is a delicate practice, and it's essential that you feel comfortable with what you are doing before you start using it on others or try to heal more substantial ailments. You've got to get used to working with the energy and moving it around in the correct way before taking on a client that has something like cancer. The main goal here is to make yourself, and others feel better. Use this skill wisely and carefully, and you shouldn't have a problem.

Finally, if you found this book useful in any way, a review on Amazon is always appreciated!

Other Books by Judith Yandell

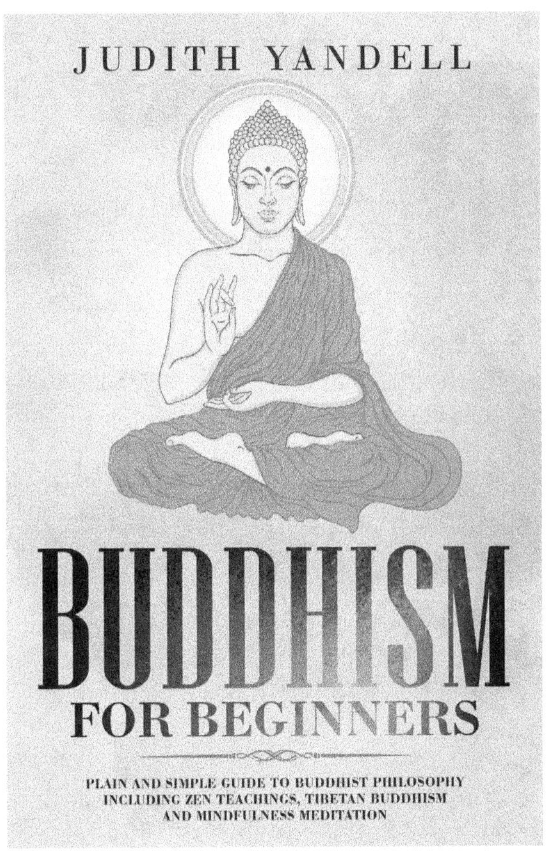

Do You Want To Free Yourself From Stress And Anxiety? Would you like to bring peace and joy in your life?

Many people hear the word "Buddhism" and they think it is a religion. However, a person of any religion can bring Buddhist principles into their life without giving up their religious beliefs.

Buddhism is a simple and practical philosophy, practiced by more than 300 million people worldwide, that can make your life better and help you find inner peace and happiness.

Buddhism is a way of living your life following a path of spiritual development that leads you to the truth of reality.

"We are shaped by our thoughts; we become what we think. When the mind is pure, joy follows like a shadow that never leaves." - Buddha

Nowadays, Buddhism is becoming increasingly popular, thanks to the positive benefits it can bring to those who choose to practice it.

By following the principles of Buddhism and by practicing mindfulness meditation you can reduce anxiety and stress and bring clarity and joy into your mind.

If you want to learn how to apply the Buddhist philosophy in your everyday life, then this book is for you.

You'll learn the principles of this philosophy along with the history of Buddha and his teachings that will help you successfully bring Buddhism into your everyday life.

This book will give you the answers you're seeking in

a format that is both simple and easy to understand, without obscure words or convoluted sentences.

Inside Buddhism for Beginners, discover:

- How you can bring peace and joy in your life following the simple principles of Buddhism
- A simple but effective meditation technique for beginners to help you relieve stress and feel calmer, even if you've never meditated before
- The core Buddhist principles and teachings explained in plain english, without complex or obscure words
- The History of Buddhism, from its origins to the present day
- Why knowing and freeing your mind can help you bring peace and joy in your everyday life (with practical tips to help you start)
- A complete historical timeline of notable buddhist events to help you understand the development of this philosophy
- The principles you should pursue if you want to follow the path of Buddha
- An effective way to understand and practice Buddhism without feeling overwhelmed
- The truth about Karma and how it can actually help you change your life (many people don't know this)
- Practical tips to bring Buddhism into your everyday life and brighten your future.
- And much, much more.

Now it's up to you. Even if right now you have no clue of Buddha's teachings, let joy and peace become part of your life and free you from stress and anxiety, you won't regret it!

"Buddhism for Beginners" by Judith Yandell is available at Amazon.

JUDITH YANDELL

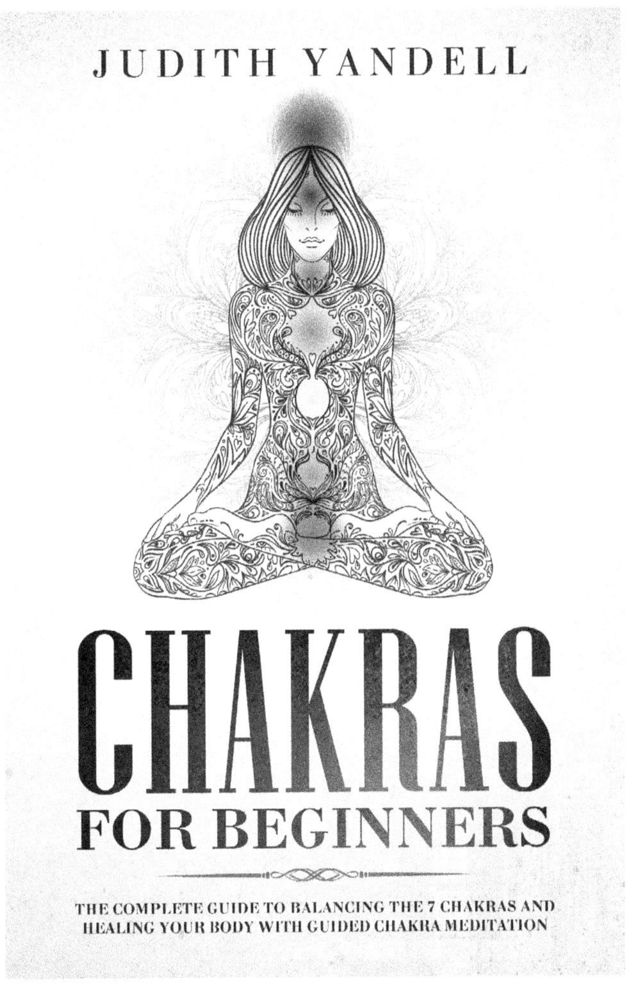

CHAKRAS
FOR BEGINNERS

THE COMPLETE GUIDE TO BALANCING THE 7 CHAKRAS AND
HEALING YOUR BODY WITH GUIDED CHAKRA MEDITATION

If you want to learn how to awaken and balance your chakras to bring joy and harmony in your life, then keep reading...

You might have a problem with your chakras without even realizing it. Do you experience headaches, neck pain or sore throat? Do you feel ill and emotionally unstable at times? Do you have troubles making decisions or feel lost and without a purpose in life? These are just a few signs of unbalanced chakras.

If you experience any of these symptoms, I want you to know that there's a solution. You see, the 7 chakras are the energy centers of your body. If they're blocked or out of balance, you'll feel the repercussions in your body. If you want to reap the benefits of a healthier mind and bring harmony in your life, you have to balance your chakras and unlock their power.

Inside Chakras for Beginners, discover:
- How you can balance your chakras and heal your energy system to bring balance into your life
- What are the 7 chakras and how do they work
- The locations and functions of the 7 chakras, from Root to Crown
- 5 lessons for clearing chakra blockages and bringing harmony and balance in your life
- How damaged chakras are affecting your life and how you can heal them (many people don't even know they have chakra blockages)
- Lists of questions to help you concentrate on the specific energy of each chakra and balance each one more effectively.
- Why balancing chakras is important and why everyone should be doing it.
- Helpful techniques and practices to keep your chakras open
- Useful strategies to bring harmony and balance in your life.
- Kundalini techniques and practices to awaken your chakras

- The most common issues created by a clogged chakra system and how to solve them
- 7 effective meditations, one for each chakra, to help you clear energy blockages and enhance your life

And much, much more!

Even if you have zero knowledge about chakras and energetic balance, this beginner's guide will help you clear your whole chakra system and live your life in harmony and balance. The truth is, when you learn how to activate and clear your chakras, they will let positive energy flow to every part of your body, mind and spirit. So, if you want to heal your body and spirit and balance your chakras to bring joy and wellness into your life, grab your copy now.

**"Chakras for Beginners" by Judith Yandell
is available at Amazon.**

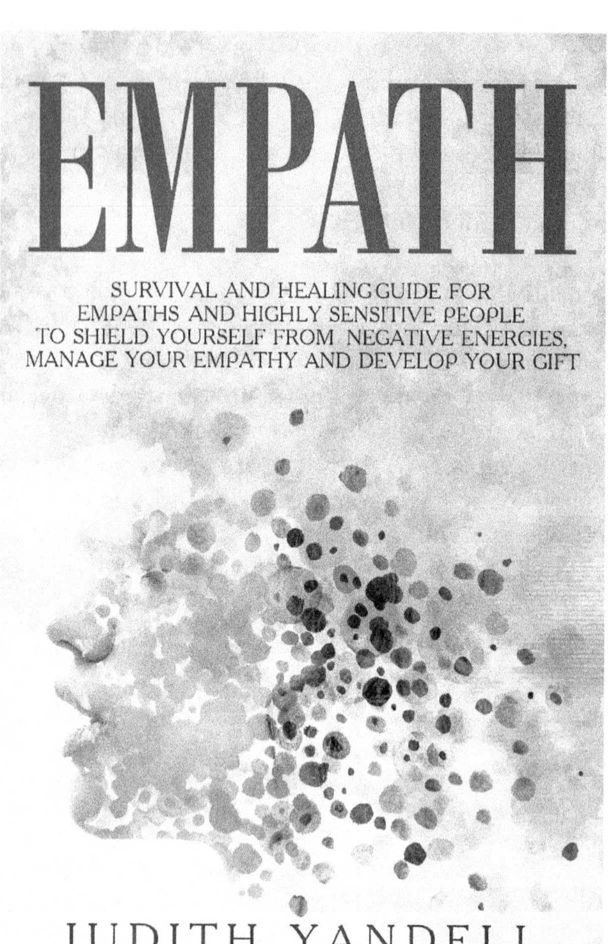

We all feel some kind of empathy towards others. But if you have no control over your empathy and always have the obsession of fixing other people, then you know how painfully frustrating being an empath is.

Empaths are usually overwhelmed by other people's emotions, they feel what others feel and are able to profoundly understand their mind. As a result, empaths care for everyone else but themselves. They become "magnets" for negative people that want to take advantage of the empaths' ability to understand opinions and emotions of others.

However, I want you to know that being an empath doesn't have to be so negative. You may have not yet realized it, but you have a powerful and beautiful gift. If you learn how to embrace it and channel your empathy, you can use it for spreading kindness, love and positive energy to the world.

In this book you'll learn:
- 6 Powerful Methods You Can Use to Control Your Gift (Hint: They Don't Include "Avoid Social Situations" and "Lock Yourself Up in You House")
- The Single Most Effective Thing You Can Do to Shield Yourself From Energy Vampires
- 11 Most Common Personality Traits of Empaths
- Powerful Techniques to Develop Your Skills and Channel Your Empathy to Spread Positive Energy
- How To Use a Specific Kind of Negative Thinking to Actually Overcome Your Social Anxiety
- 20 Statements to Help You Determine if You Really Are an Empath
- Is an Energy Vampire Preying on You? Here's How to Find Out
- How to Find Out if Your Child Is an Empath and What You Can Do to Support
- A Positive Affirmations Routine That Can Help You Accept Yourself as an Empath and Strengthen Your Abilities
- How Detoxifying a Certain Area of Your Brain Can Help You Embrace Your Empathic Abilities and

Improve Your Sense of Intuition
- Why in Certain Cases Accepting Negativity Can Actually Help You Feel Better.

Even if right now you feel you have no control over your abilities, I want you to know that you can learn how to manage your empathy and develop your gift in the right way.

**"Empath" by Judith Yandell
is available at Amazon.**